DR. PIERRE F. WALTER

ALTERNATIVE MEDICINE AND WELLNESS TECHNIQUES

14 Pathways to Integral Health

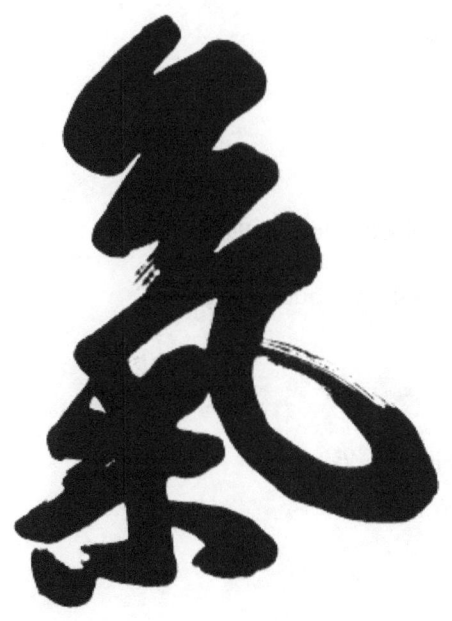

"Scholarly Articles Series"

Published by Sirius-C Media Galaxy LLC

http://sirius-c-publishing.com

http://siriuscmedia.com

http://ipublica.com

ISBN 978-1-466461-80-2

Contact Information Dr. Pierre F. Walter

publisher@sirius-c-publishing.com

About Pierre F. Walter

http://drpfw.info

Quotation Suggestion

Pierre F. Walter, *Alternative Medicine and Wellness Techniques: 14 Pathways to Integral Health,* Newark: Sirius-C Media Galaxy LLC, 2011

About the Author

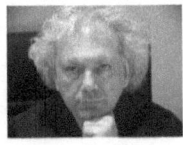

Pierre F. Walter is an author, international lawyer, researcher, corporate trainer, and lecturer. After finalizing studies in German Law, International Law and *European integration* with diplomas obtained in 1981 through 1983, he graduated in December 1987 at the Law Faculty of the University of Geneva as *Docteur en Droit* in international law.

The doctorate was funded by scholarships from the *Swiss Institute of Comparative Law*, Lausanne, and from the *University of Geneva*, as well as a Fulbright Travel Grant for an assistantship with Professor Louis B. Sohn at *UGA Law School Department of International Law*, Athens, Georgia, USA, in 1985. Pierre F. Walter also served as a research assistant to *Freshfields, Bruckhaus, Deringer,* Cologne, Germany in 1983 and to *Lalive Lawyers*, Geneva, in 1987.

Pierre F. Walter writes and lectures in English, German and French languages; he has written *more than ten thousand pages* embracing all literary genres, including *novels, short stories, film scripts, essays, selfhelp books, monographs* and extended *book reviews*. Also a pianist and composer, he has realized 40 CDs with *jazz, newage* and *relaxation music.*

Pierre F. Walter's professional publications span the domains *International Law, Criminal Law, Holistic Science, Psychology, Education, Shamanism, Ecology, Spirituality, Quantum Physics, Systems Theory, Natural Healing, Peace Research, Personal Growth, Selfhelp* and *Consciousness Research*. 110 Book Reviews, thirty-eight audio books and more than hundred video lectures were realized in the years 2005-2010. Besides, Pierre F. Walter is author and editor of *Great Minds Series*, which features scientists, artists and authors of genius from Leonardo to Fritjof Capra and of 'Scholarly Articles Series'.

Pierre F. Walter publishes via his Delaware firm *Sirius-C Media Galaxy LLC* and the imprints IPUBLICA and Sirius-C Media (SCM).

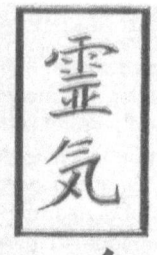

Reiki

USUI SHIKI RYOHO

This is to certify that

Pierre Frederic Walter

has completed

the First Degree in the

Usui System of Natural Healing

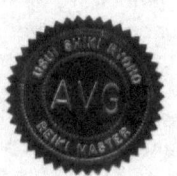

Rotterdam 4-10-'94

Anneke van Gelder

Master

Phyllis Lei Furumoto

Grand Master
The Reiki Alliance

REIKI

THIS SERVES TO CERTIFY THAT

Peter Fritz Walter.

HAS RECEIVED THE USUI-TIBETAN SYSTEM OF ATTUNEMENT AND TRAINING FOR THE

SECOND DEGREE

---

15 July 1999

DATE

Chandra Naidu.

REIKI MASTER
SOUTH AFRICA

CONTENTS

NATUROPATHY

An American Natural Healing System

The Six Principles of Healing

Nature's Healing Power

Identify the Cause

Do No Harm

Whole Person Treatment

The Physician is Teacher

Disease Prevention

OSTEOPATHY

The Eight Principles of Osteopathic Healing

What is Osteopathy?

The Eight Principles of Osteopathy

QIGONG

The Art of Breathing

What is Qigong?

The Qigong Posture

Qigong for Healing Sadism

RADIONICS

The Unknown Medical Science

Tai Chi Chuan, by Master Shou-Yu Liang

The path of initiation is branded in the West as degenerate; by contrast, in tribal society the initiation of the shaman is accepted, even encouraged and supported by everyone; and the teacher helps the student to decipher his experiences by means of cultural symbols. But in our culture the symbols of transformation are negative: they include hospitalization, schizophrenia, brain-wave tests, stupefying psychotropic drugs, and ostracism from society. How many unrecognized shamans, mediums, and saints fill the madhouses of rationalism? How many powers have been mangled and cut off during the long history of psychiatry? How many people has psychology reduced to mindless robots through its abasement of the psyche? The spiritual climate in our society shuts down shamanic experience in its incipient stages, distorts it and desacralizes it as neurosis and psychotic deception. But psychic transformation cannot be extirpated by societal taboos. Spiritual experience is a transhistorical, transcultural phenomenon and can break through in individuals at any time.
– Holger Kalweit, *Shamans, Healers and Medicine Men*, Boston: Shambhala, 2000, p. 54

OVERVIEW

The 14 Ways to Wellness

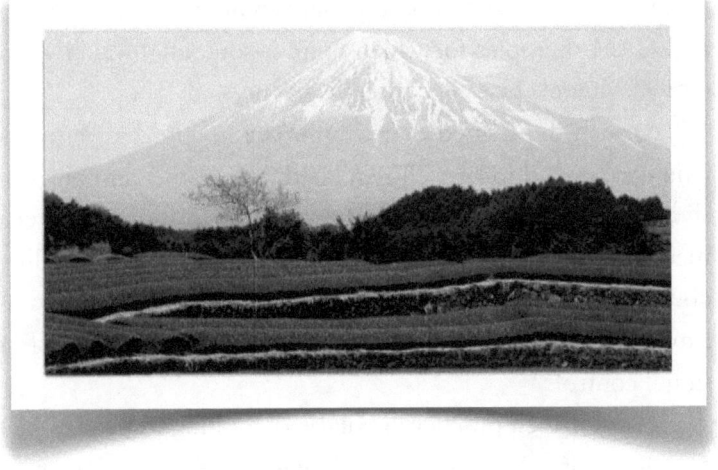

Alternative Medicine in the United States

For the United States, *The National Center for Complementary and Alternative Medicine* defines complementary and alternative medicine as a group of diverse medical and health care systems, practices, and products that are not presently considered to be part of conventional medicine. It also defines integrative medicine as combining mainstream medical therapies and CAM therapies for which there is some high-quality scientific evidence of safety and effectiveness.

As such the United States' approach to alternative medicine can be said to be well-regulated, integrative and permissive to practices that may not be part of traditional Western medicine. The regulations in place are focused upon avoiding abusive and incompetent practices and outright charlatanism, through a system of minimum requirements and professional control.

The fourteen practices I will be describing in this booklet are all regulated in the United States, while regulations may differ from state to state. But they are recognized as valid alternative medical practices.

The Fourteen Practices

Ayurveda

Ayurveda is India's oldest indigenous medical science. It is completely non-chemical and non-harmful, and highly effective. It has been promoted by Mahatma Gandhi and came to be known in the West through his writings and the British colonization of India.

Chinese Medicine

Chinese medicine and pharmacology is based on the natural flow of the *ch'i*, the bioplasmatic energy that I came to call *e-force* and that is an angular stone in the ancient Chinese system of healing illness.

Homeopathy

Homeopathy was founded by Samuel Hahnemann, and was expanded very importantly by Edward Bach.

Kirlian Photography

Kirlian Photography refers to a form of contact print photography, theoretically associated with high-voltage. It is named after the Russian physician, Dr. Semyon Kirlian, who in 1939 discovered that if an object on a photographic plate is subjected to a strong electric field, an image is created on the plate.

Kyodo

Kyudo, literally meaning way of the bow, is the Japanese art of archery. It is a modern Japanese martial art *(gendai budo)*. It is estimated that there are approximately half a million practitioners of Kyodo today.

Naturopathy

Naturopathy is a natural healing practice that is genuinely American and taught at major natural healing centers and universities in California, Arizona and Texas. While it may be taught elsewhere at reputed universities in the United States, the centers and universities in the three mentioned states are the most recognized. This has historical and climatic reasons. The plants used in naturopathy best grow in the hotter climatic regions of the North American belt.

Osteopathy

Osteopathy is equally a natural healing practice that originates from the United States.

Qigong

Qigong, or *ch'i kung*, refers to a wide variety of traditional cultivation practices that involve methods of accumulating, circulating, and working with *ch'i*, breathing or energy within the body. Qigong is practiced for health maintenance purposes, as a therapeutic intervention, as a medical profession, a spiritual path and/or component of Chinese martial arts.

Radionics

Radionics is a science that to this day is understood only by a few, as it is so far still largely located within the gray area between official science and spirituality, unknown to the great public. But that does not diminish its importance. It owns its existence to two rather distinct streams of influence, for one the esoteric spiritual teachings of Alice Bailey, on one hand, and the experimental findings of the Russian-French scientist Georges Lakhovsky, on the other.

Reiki

Reiki is a spiritual practice developed in 1922 by Mikao Usui. After three weeks of fasting and meditating on Mount Kurama, in Japan, Usui claimed to receive the ability of healing without energy depletion. A portion of the practice, *tenohira* or palm healing, is used as a form of complementary and alternative medicine (CAM). Tenohira is a technique whereby practitioners believe they are moving healing energy (a form of *ki*) through the palms.

Sophrology

Sophrology was created by Dr. Alfonso Caycedo in the 1960s. It is a branch of mindbody psychology that focuses on understanding human consciousness and altered states of consciousness for short-term or long-term positive modifications, relaxation and purposes of personal growth and creativity boosting. The term is derived from old Greek and means *study of the harmony of consciousness.*

Tai Chi Chuan

Tai Chi Chuan is an internal Chinese martial art, often promoted and practiced as a martial arts therapy for the purposes of health and longevity. Tai Chi Chuan is considered a soft style martial art, an art applied with as much deep relaxation or softness in the musculature as possible, to distinguish its theory and application from that of the hard martial art styles which use a degree of tension in the muscles.

Tibetan Medicine

Tibetan Medicine is one of the most ancient natural healing traditions in the world. Much of it is not yet known in the West. I know little about it, except that Tibetan doctors are the most trained in pulse reading and can predict diseases years ahead. So on this page I just report a personal experience.

Yoga

The Sanskrit word *Yoga* means to join or unite. It is generally translated as union of the individual atman or individual soul with paramatman or universal soul.

Yoga is a family of ancient spiritual practices dating back more than 5000 years from India. It is one of the six schools of Hindu philosophy.

Why Did I Write this Guide?

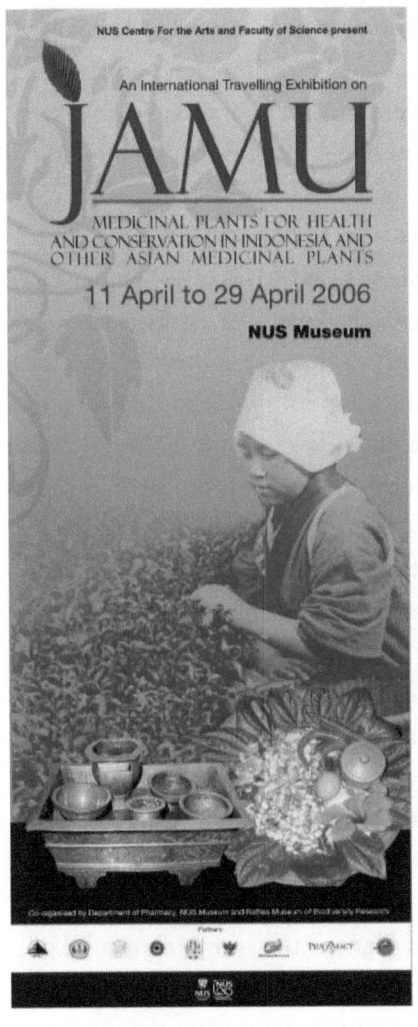

Let me elucidate shortly why I came to write this little guide. It was not out of sheer curiosity, nor for attracting readers to my rather voluminous book collection. Instead, my *primary motivation* was that during all of my childhood and youth, not only myself, but also my mother, grandmother, and later my wife were to suffer *medical malpractice.* I can say with conviction that my mother had lived at least ten years longer, had she not trusted the ignorance of the gods in white coats, or what I came to call '*international medical business*'. My wife was almost killed by a doctor who had performed a spinal punctation with local anesthesia, for which it is absolutely paramount that the patient be in a *horizontal posi-*

tion for at least twenty-four hours, without interruption. What the doctor did was to send my wife home after a few hours. The result was that she had to be hospitalized as she was almost dying from the headaches and other consequences of this very dangerous intervention. I was interviewing several doctors in our local hospital about her case and one of them was scandalized and said that the operation had been a clear case of medical malpractice.

But a moment later, when I said I was a law student and intended to sue that doctor for medical malpractice, and wanted him to testify in court against his colleague, he waved me off, saying I had 'misunderstood' him and that he could not allege anything of that kind. Two minutes later I was out of the office. Needless to add that he had not invited me to come back.

I became aware what a sordid club this modern medicine was, how false and sworn into stubborn resistance they were, and I began to understand that they had indeed much to lose and much to defend, that namely their whole brilliant empire was built on very shaky ground.

I came to see clearly that they have no idea what really causes disease, and what most upset me was how sluggishly most doctors handle their obligation to have the patient's full consent for any treatment they engage. In practice namely, in most cases they take it for granted that the patient consents or they get a consent, but not an informed one because they have not completely informed the patient what the treatment really incurs, short term, and in the long run.

After all, my mother was virtually killed by those doctors in the Catholic hospital where she was constantly maltreated and sadly died at an age when she did not need to, only because the doctors did not recognize the psychic condition of her heart disease and virtually massacred her, by one operation after the other, until her heart was stuffed with metal machinery – that her body eventually rejected!

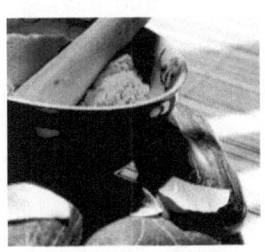 These shortcomings got me to be interested in *alternative medicine* from about my thirties. I first had the opportunity to study Reiki with Anneke van Gelder, a *Reiki Master* from Holland, acquiring the first degree, then, five years later, with Chandra Naidu from South Africa, acquiring the second degree or initiation in the Usui alternative healing system. The third, and most important initiation, which results in the title of *Reiki Master*, was offered to me by Ugo di Marino, an Italian *Reiki Master*, in Bali, in 2000, but I refused to receive it, as I felt I was not ready.

Ugo had waived the twenty thousand dollars fee that is obligatory for receiving this title, and I didn't find it correct to receive the title without giving 'money energy' back for the energy received. In addition, I felt I wasn't dedicated enough, at that time, distracted by a quite important business project. But this *Reiki Master* told me I had all the capacities of a true master in this art of energy healing.

But the most important feedback, I got from Anneke, back in 1994, when I started out with my Reiki practice. Anneke had quite a number of students, and a thriving practice, with patients from the middle and upper classes in Rotterdam. Anneke was a very gifted healer; she was able to do distance healing as well. Some of her patients were Americans whom she treated over the phone, at any time of the day or the night, as the client found it convenient.

Now for me, as I never had done any healing practice and had no idea I had a talent for it, it was important was Anneke could sense when I treated her, after having learnt the basics. And surprisingly so, Anneke said I was an exceptional student, that she never had somebody with just beginner knowledge who had such a powerful aura. Only later was I informed by potential astrology that, besides having Sun in the 6th House, which is the quintessential 'healer' positioning of the Sun in a birth chart, I was having quite a few constellations in my chart that were pointing to my talent for healing and my strong luminous energy field. Finally, between 1998 and 2000, being a member of the *Parapsychological Association* of Jakarta, Indonesia, I was screened by several first rate psychics who fully confirmed what Anneke had told me.

The psychics said that my human energy field was exceptionally strong and powerful and that I should use it for healing others.

And a test was made. Several boys who had been circumcised were taken to me for treatment and the results were convincing and surprising everybody, including the boys' fathers who were attending the healing session. What I did was simply to hold both of my hands over the penis of each boy, about half an hour, ejecting energy from my palms, which was felt by the boys as 'warm and nice'. One boy was dreadfully maltreated by the quack who had cut his foreskin. He was still bleeding after one week and his penis looked painfully distorted. It was all inflammated and the boy, according to what his father said, suffered from his condition more than any other boy. He suffered atrocious pain when urinating.

This boy I treated twice, on two consecutive mornings, each time for about one hour, and the results were miraculous. After the first treatment, the boy was pain-free and could urinate without pain. And the bleeding stopped right after the treatment. After the second treatment, the boy smiled, for the first time, and said:

– I feel good now, I think it's all good.

After my long stay in Indonesia, I was suffering from an ongoing diarrhea and upon returning back to Germany, I was seeing a *Reiki Master*. She had been initiated by powerful Filipino healers in the Philippines. Again, I got to hear I had been the victim of medical malpractice because the diagnosis by her husband, a medical doctor, revealed that my intestinal flora was completely gone. The doctor was scandalized, saying:

– You have no more bacteria in your intestines, so how is your body going to digest any food? It's impossible. We have to rebuild your intestinal flora, and that will take some time. Until then, you need to be on a strict diet.

I had been consulting Western doctors in Jakarta who had given me huge amounts of antibiotics, and as my condition was recurring, I took those antibiotics almost for one whole year.

My condition was healed completely, and only through homeopathy, Bach Flowers and Reiki, and later on, upon returning to Asia, with Chinese herbal concoctions.

And the third motivational factor, then, for my research on alternative medicine and wellness techniques was what I was learning about native healing in Indonesia first, and then, a few years later in Vietnam and Cambodia. When I first arrived in Yogyakarta, back in 1996, I remember to have counted between 120 and 150 shops and streets kiosks that

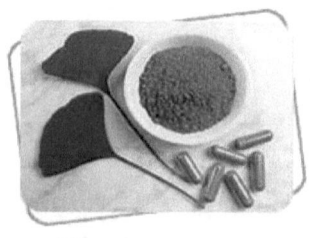

were selling the age-old *Jamu* plant medicine, and related homeopathic products of which the local culture in Java used to be so rich.

Jamu is a yellow powder that is won from grinding the roots of certain trees. This powder, then, is mixed with hot water and the yellow of an egg, and this gives a cup of delicious brew that heals about everything.

There were more than one hundred different Jamu concoctions in one of the larger shops. The street kiosks were selling between five and twenty of them, sufficient for the common ailments such as 'sakit panas' (fever), 'diare' (diarrhea), or 'anak-anak panas' (child fever). In fact, fever is a severe and very dangerous condition in Java and also in Bali. I have spoken to a young man who lost his two small children in one night. The fever was shooting up so quickly that every help was too late. Two children of one and two years died and left behind a couple in deep and lasting depression.

Of course, in such a case, Western medicine could have helped effectively, but the man was very poor and I am not sure he could have afforded to pay the hospital.

Two years later, I was shocked to see that only about ten to twenty of those shops and kiosks remained, and a year later, in 1999, I was counting just five. Why had all the others disappeared? Because of Western medicine suddenly being recognized as 'better' and 'cleaner', and so on and so forth, through television and USA-driven publicity. It appeared that only people in the countryside, and elders, were keeping true to their traditional medicine.

The problem is complex. Pharmacies I saw in Indonesia, Vietnam and Cambodia sell Western pharmaceutical products like bread, without any product knowledge, and any restriction. All can be bought that is in-store, no prescription needed. As these locals cannot read the leaflets, they have hardly any knowledge about the particular pharmaceuticals, and their side-effects and dangers. I have seen in several shops *Valium 20* that since decades is legally forbidden in Europe, huge pills, sold to a teenager. The prices are much higher compared to the very cheap Jamu concoctions. Jamu typically was sold for about ten cent per concoction, while for most medicines, it's a few dollars each.

So there are *two problem complexes* interwoven with each other. The first is lack of knowledge. While the Jamu sellers had excellent knowledge of their products, this is seldom the case with modern-day pharmacies, in these countries. The second problem is the financial hurdle, as modern pharmacy virtually bleeds the locals out, who in urgent cases take exorbitant credits with village usurers, for which they pay *between twenty and sixty percent* of monthly (not yearly) interest!

With hospitals, it's the same. In Cambodia, when somebody has not enough money to pay the doctor upon arrival in the hospital, the person is not treated. I have heard many stories of people who died virtually under the eyes of doctors because they had not enough money to pay for an urgency operation. So they were not treated. A Vietnamese friend of mine in Cambodia was having an unwanted pregnancy but did not opt for abortion. When the baby was on the point to come out, she quickly went to a hospital and called me on my handphone to send her two hundred dollars for paying the doctor. I replied that it was okay and that I was sending the money with my driver, who however came to be stuck in a traffic jam. The doctor refused to help the baby to leave the womb as the money had not arrived in time, and the baby died in the womb and had to be removed surgically. The doctor cashed the two hundred dollars in for giving birth to a dead fetus.

Another consequence of medical costs, that is even uglier than this story, is a fact that was reported to me by several trustworthy university graduates. In Cambodia, when a person is injured by a traffic accident, the hospital costs might be outrageous for a local person who has caused the accident. The simple and brutal consequence is that victims are killed and those who are guilty of causing the accident take it and leave it.

In one case, witnessed by a friend of mine, a trustworthy business graduate, a truck driver had collided with a motorcycle, and the heavily injured and bleeding woman who drove the motorcycle was screaming, on the floor, a few meters in front of the truck. The driver did not think long, restarted the motor, drove right over the screaming victim, and took flight. When police and ambulance arrived, every help was too late. I was being told that this happens in Phnom Penh virtually every day. The reason is not a particular murderous instinct in Cambodian people, but the outrageous hospital costs and absence of any obligatory national insurance.

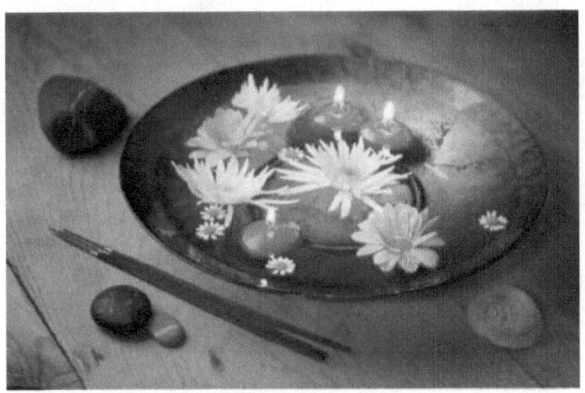

I recently had my maid's uncle being hospitalized for a stroke. The doctors didn't do anything as the family is very poor. The moment they knew I was willing to pay, several doctors came to examine the man. Subsequently, an x-ray was proposed that was quoted to me with two hundred dollars while locals normally pay between twenty and thirty dollars for the same x-ray. It's all a question of money, the whole medical business, and that is why I call it so. *It is a business, and*

nothing but a business! And its objective is *not healing,* but money-making. It is significant that for Western doctors, the expression 'healer' is an insult. They should be called medical business consultants, or pharmaceutical sales agents, not doctors, for that's what they are.

These are some of the ugly consequences of Western medical business reaching Asia for 'saving many human lives through our enlightened Western medicine'. It's just on the same line as Western sex morality reaching Asia for 'cutting down on child prostitution'. The results in that other war for 'spreading enlightened Western morality and democracy around the world' are even uglier, as I report them in the *Idiot Guide to World Peace (2010).*

AYURVEDA

The Science of Life

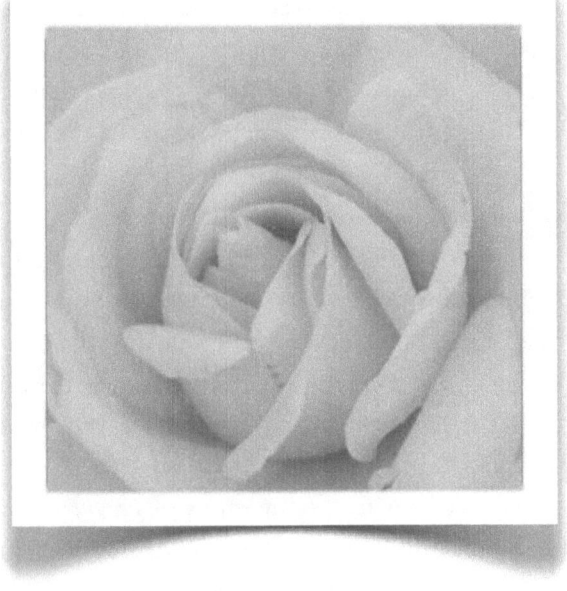

Introduction

I was becoming aware of Ayurveda when, back in the 1970s, I was reading Gandhi. Gandhi was often reporting in his writings that he put his faith not in modern medicine but in age-old Ayurveda and that he had healed all his ailments with the simple recipes for healthy living that Ayurveda teaches as a matter of prophylaxis. I was intrigued and bought a book about Ayurveda and the information resonated deeply in my soul. I found many of the Ayurveda precepts very similar to what I had learnt about Chinese and Tibetan Medicine.

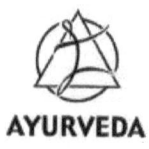

AYURVEDA

The name *Ayurveda* is significant as it means something like *Life Knowledge* or *Science of Life* – and there is about no greater gap to traditional Western medicine which could be called *Science of Death* because it gained knowledge not from observing the living changes in life's texture, but by vivisecting cadavers.

Ayurveda deals with the measures of *healthy living*, along with therapeutic measures that relate to physical, mental, social and spiritual harmony. Ayurveda is also one among the few traditional systems of medicine involving surgery.

Ayurveda is a wholeness and wellness approach to medicine which means that *its concepts are holistic* and consider life as a dynamic process. It avoids any harsh and especially irrevocable treatments and favors *soft remedies* such as plant concoctions, and massage.

An Ayurveda Experience

On a trip to India back in 2006, I was having Ayurveda treatments in a reputed *Ayurveda Clinic* in Trivandrum, Kerala. I got daily massage with warm oil, which is a wonderful therapy that relaxed me deeply. After the first treatments, before I got used to it, I was so completely relaxed and put at rest, that upon coming back to the hotel, I had to sleep for the whole afternoon.

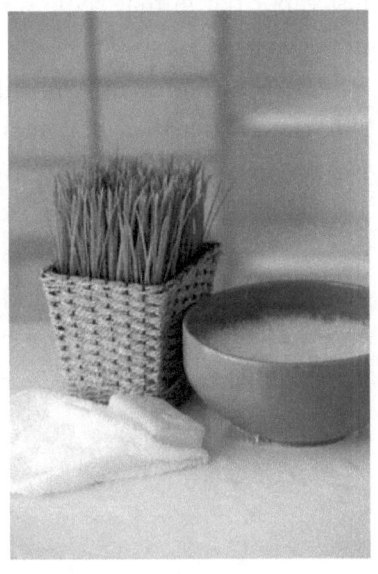

One day, I took an additional treatment, thus after the massage, that they call steam bath, but it's not like a steam sauna at all. You are sitting in a wooden container to which a tube is connected that transports the hot vapor. The casing is closed around you and there is a rubber ring around your neck that prevents steam from getting out. So your face and head are cold while your body gets very hot, and that is a wise idea.

I was sitting in that wooden box, on a little chair, and saw in front of me a stove on which a water kettle was boiling. From the top of the kettle there was that tube leading right to a pipe system that borders the bottom of the box. There are many little holes in these pipes from which the vapor streams into the box. You really get hot there, but gradually, and after fifteen minutes, just at the right moment, they liberate you from this sweating experience. And the surprise was that that day, when I came back to the hotel, I was not tired at all. I never knew that a steam bath can revitalize you to that extent. And yes, I forgot to mention the most important. It's not just vapor but in that kettle were a lot of fresh herbs boiling in the water …

Then I went to an Ayurveda doctor and got some medicine against diarrhea and another one for my swelling legs. But unfortunately I had to leave the whole plastic bag at the airport in Trivandrum because they really take flight safety serious in India, to a point to annoy you, and only one bag is allowed to take on-board, and I had already two with me, and my suitcase was full to a breaking point …, so I had to leave all that wonderful medicine behind in India.

CHINESE MEDICINE

Another Life Science

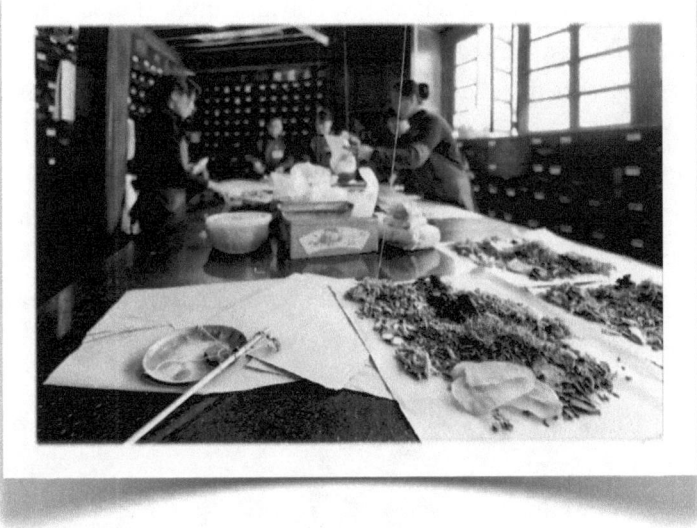

Introduction

Traditional Chinese medicine is a range of traditional medical practices used in China that developed over several thousand years. These practices include herbal medicine, acupuncture, and massage.

Other East Asian medical systems, such as traditional Japanese, Korean or Tibetan medicine, apply similar principles. Chinese medicine was perhaps the first really *holistic* medicine on the globe, and it sees processes of the human body as interrelated and constantly interacting energetically with the environment.

Chinese medicine recognizes that good health is basically a state of harmony and therefore looks for the *signs of disharmony* in the external and internal environment of a person in order to understand, treat and prevent disease.

It was back in the 1980s that I got to learn about Chinese Medicine for the first time. I was reading several books about it and discovered a truly holistic approach 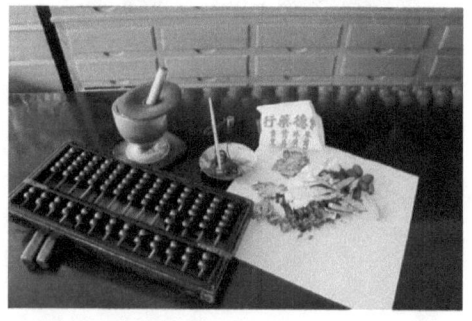 to health, something completely unknown until this day to palliative and symptom-focused Western 'business' medicine.

As I set out to study it more in detail, I found, in 1995, a CD-ROM produced by Hopkins University with the title

Traditional Chinese Medicine and Pharmacology, from which I will provide some quotes here. The author is the Director of the All-China Association of Traditional Chinese Medicine and Advisor to the Public Health Ministry of the People's Republic of China, Professor Don Jianhua.

This opened me doors to a more thorough understanding of the particular approach of Chinese traditional medicine to restoring health as well as to disease prevention. There is namely a much stronger focus in Chinese medicine upon *disease prevention* as this is the case in Western medicine.

Professor Don Jianhua

The basic theories of traditional Chinese medicine describe the physiology and pathology of the human body, disease etiology, diagnosis, and differentiation of symptom-complexes. This includes the theories of Yin-Yang, Five Elements, zang-fu, channels-collaterals, qi, blood, body fluid, methods of diagnosis, and differentiation of symptom-complexes.

Traditional Chinese medical theories possess two outstanding features, their holistic point of view, and their application of treatment according to the differentiation of symptom-complexes. According to these traditional viewpoints, the zang-fu organs are the core of the human body as an organic entity in which tissues and sense organs are connected through a network of channels and collaterals. This concept is applied extensively to physiology, pathology, diagnosis, and treatment.

The functional physiological activities of the zang-fu organs are dissimilar, but they work in coordination. There exists an organic connection between the organs and their related tissues. Pathologically, a dysfunction of the zang-fu organs may be reflected on the body surface through the channels and their collaterals. At the same time, diseases of body surface tissues may also affect their related zang or fu organs. Affected zang or fu organs may also influence each other through internal connections. Traditional Chinese medical treatment consists of regulating the functions of the zang-fu organs in order to correct pathological changes. With acupuncture, treatment is accomplished by stimulating certain areas of the external body.

Not only is the human body an organic whole, but it is also a unified entity within nature, so changes in the natural environment may directly or indirectly affect it. For example, changes of the four seasons, and the alternations of day and night may change the functional condition of the human body, while various geographical environments can influence differences in body constitution, and so on. These factors must be considered when diagnosis and treatment are given. The principles of treatment are expected to accord with the different seasons and environments.

Application of treatment according to the differentiation of syndromes is another characteristic of traditional Chinese medicine. 'Differentiation of syndromes' means to analyze the disease condition in order to know its essentials, to identify the causative facts, the location and nature, and to obtain conclusions about the confrontation between pathogenic and antipathogenic factors. In traditional Chinese medicine, differentiation performed to outline the specific principles and methods of treatment because similar diseases may have different clinical manifestations, while different diseases may share the same syndromes.

Treatment in traditional Chinese medicine stresses the differences of syndromes, but not the differences of diseases. Therefore different treatments for the same disease exist and different diseases can be treated by the same method.

Copyright 2005 Hopkins Technology.

Yin & Yang

The primordial energy, when working on the earth plane, manifests in dualistic form, as two complementary energies, *Yin and Yang*. Both of the energies can be associated with certain characteristics. *Yin* can be associated with the female principle; this does however not mean that it is identical with it. We talk about corresponding characteristics or elements, and the system as such is one of corresponding relationships. Accordingly, *yin* can be said to correspond with water, the female principle, the color black, the direction down or a landscape that is flat. *Yang* can be said to correspond with fire, the male principle, the color white, the direction up or with a landscape that is mountainous. In every *yin* there is a bit of *yang*, and in every *yang* a bit of *yin*. This bit is the essence that is multiplied once the point of culmination has been passed.

Professor Don Jianhua

Yin and yang represent two opposite aspects of every object an dits implicit conflict and interdependence. Generally, anything that is moving, ascending, bright, progressing, hyperactive, including functional disease of the body, pertains to yang. The characteristics of stillness, descending, darkness, degeneration, hypoactivity, including organic disease, pertain to yin.

The nature of yin and yang is relative. According to Yin-Yang theory, everything in the universe can be divided into the two opposite but complementary aspects of yin and yang and so on ad infinitum. For example, day is yang and night is yin, but morning is understood as being yang within yang, afternoon is yin within yang, evening before midnight is yin within yin and the time after midnight is yang within yin.

What that means is that for example *yin* moves towards its fullness in order to culminate and swap its nature into *yang*. *Yang*, when it culminates, becomes *yin*. That is why we can say change is programmed into the very essence of the *yin-yang* dualism and thus, change cannot be avoided. We can even go as far as saying that the very fact of change is the proof that we deal with a living thing. If there is no change, there is no movement and, as a result, no life. Life is change, living movement.

The *yin-yang* duality principle is very far-reaching. It also encompasses the art of cooking. The Tao of cooking prescribes that every dish should be composed in a way to balance *yin* and *yang* and the four tastes sweet, salty, sour and bitter. Every vegetable, every kind of meat or fish, and every other food has been qualified by the sages of old to be either *yin* or *yang*.

This knowledge forms an essential part of the Chinese system of health care and of the martial arts, which can be expressed in the slogan 'food is medicine'.

Professor Don Jianhua

The yin and yang aspects within an object are not quiescent, but in a state of constant motion. They can be described as being in a state where the lessening of yin leads to an increase of yang, or vice versa. (...)

Regarding the human body's functional activities, which are considered yang, the consumption of nutrient substances which are considered yin, results in the lessening of yin to the increase of yang. As the metabolism of nutrient substances (yin) exhausts the functional energy (yang) to a certain extent, this is understood as a lessening of yang to the increase of yin.

> Under normal conditions the mutual consuming and increasing of yin and yang maintain a relative balance. Under abnormal conditions there is an excess or insufficiency of either yin or yang which leads to the occurrence of disease.
>
> Copyright 2005 Hopkins Technology.

In the martial arts, the same principle applies. The beginner of learning the art of Kung Fu is developing consciousness. And second breathing. The right way of breathing stresses that we exhale on the effort. It is not the muscles that do exceptional things, but breath or *prana*. In Kung Fu exercises the perfection of the movements is impossible to achieve if the breathing technique is wrong. You can even say that the movements have no value in themselves besides forcing us to breathe correctly. By balancing *yin* and *yang* in our mindbody, the very source of our being, the Tao within us becomes activated and can more easily guide us and enrich us from inside. It is our true power. But without balancing *yin* and *yang* in our mindbody, its power is spoilt by the many negative influences that modern life inflicts upon it.

Our emotions, like all in life, are reigned by the *duality principle,* they ebb up and they flow down, they increase and they decrease, and eventually they go through a culmination point and then change. Let me demonstrate this again with an example. When you are enraged, your rage will increase until it reaches a culmination point. What happens when it reaches this point? The astonishing thing is that you will not experience lesser rage then, but no rage at all!

Your rage will change into another emotion, for example joy, or it will completely cease with no other emotion overtaking: you are at peace.

Why is that so? This is so because all our emotions are interconnected in what I call a *kaleidoscopic succession*. A kaleidoscope is a device where the prism is split off by a lens into its basic spectral colors. These devices that many of us know from our childhood, are designed like little photographic cameras or glasses and you could look at any object using the kaleidoscope as a filter. You would then see life in many different colorful shades. This metaphor fits emotions very well.

Our emotions are the basic spectral colors of the light beam of life which is like a bundled beam of white light. Every emotion, by the frequency of the spectral color that it adds on to the beam of the bioenergy, completes the white beam. As you know from optics, light can only be white if the spectrum is complete. And so it is with our emotions. Your vital energies are only complete and strong if all your emotions are active and contribute their specific bioelectric frequencies to the main frequency of the bioenergy that flows through your organism. When you block one of the emotions, that part of the frequency is lacking or becomes distorted.

As a result, your white beam of vital energy will not be really white anymore and thus will be weakened. That is why the duality of our emotions is so important and must be functional if emotions are to flow healthily.

Now, let us see who this interrelatedness and mutual transformation of yin and yang which could also be called the 'dualistic principle' works in the holistic treatment of disease.

Professor Don Jianhua

The mutual transformation of yin and yang is often seen during the development of a disease. For example, if a patient has a constant high fever, which is suddenly lowered, accompanied by a pale complexion, cold limbs, extremely feeble pulse (the danger symptoms of yin cold syndromes), we may say that the disease has transformed from a yang syndrome into a yin syndrome. Under these circumstances, proper emergency treatment should warm the limbs to make the pulse normal. The yang qi will recover, and the danger will be removed. Thus yin syndromes can change into yang syndromes. (...)

For example, the activities (yang) of a particular organ are based on that organ's substance (yin) and when either of these aspects are absent, the other cannot function. Thus the result of physiological activities is to constantly promote the transformation of yang into yin essence. If yin and yang cannot maintain relative balance and interaction, they will separate from each other ending the life that depends on them. (...)

In medical treatment, the theory of yin and yang is not only used to decide the principles of treatment. This theory is also generally applied to the properties, flavor and action of Chinese herbal medicine as a guide to the clinical administration of herbs. For example, drugs with cold, cool or moist properties are classified as yin and drugs with the opposite properties are classified as yang. Herbs with sour, bitter, or salty flavors are yin, while those with pungent, sweet, or insipid flavors are yang. Drugs with an astringent or descending action are yin and those with an ascending and dispersing action are yang. In clinical treatment, we should determine the principles of treatment based on an analysis of the yin and yang conditions present in terms of their different yin-yang properties and actions. The goal of clinical treatment is to restore the healthy yin-yang properties and actions to restore a healthy yin-yang balance in the patient.

The Five Elements

The principle of the five elements suggests that nature is *interactive* and in a continuous process of transformation. The five elements wood, fire, water, earth and metal are mutually constructive and also mutually destructive. For example, wood is positively enhanced by water whereas water destroys fire. These two parallel processes of creation and destruction can be seen as two circles or cycles, a *cycle of creation*, and a *cycle of destruction*.

Professor Don Jianhua

The Five Elements theory posits wood, fire, earth, metal, and water as the basic elements of the material world. These elements are in constant movement and change. Moreover, the complex connections between material objects are explained through the relationship of interdependence and mutual restraint that governs the five elements. In traditional Chinese medicine Five Elements Theory is used to interpret the relationship between the physiology and pathology of the human body and the natural environment.

Copyright 2005 Hopkins Technology.

The principle of the five elements teaches us that nothing in nature is static or stagnant, but that all is subject to continuous flow, continuous change. It also teaches us that all elements naturally interact with each other, mutually depend on each other, and that nothing is really isolated. As a result, we can verify if our understanding of nature is in accordance with the laws of nature.

Studying and observing these laws, we notice a high degree of *interdependence* in nature and a high *interactivity*, a fact that in the Western sciences has only recently been given the focus it deserves. It is modern systems theory that deals with the interactive processes in nature.

The principle of the *five elements*, as simplistic as it may seem on first sight, is a wonderful teacher of real-life functions that can help us to correct our way to see the world, ourselves and others and to more accurately evaluate the impact that every single of our actions might have on life as a whole. It is the point of departure of a holistic view of life.

Professor Don Jianhua

The Five Elements theory is applied to the physiology and pathology of the human body by using the relationship of generation and subjugation to guide clinical diagnosis and treatment. (…)

Physiologically the Five Elements theory explains the unity of the mutual relationships between the zang-fu organs and body tissues as well as between the human body and nature. The physiological activities of the five zang organs can be classified according to the different characteristics of the five elements. For example, the liver is said to preside over the vigorous flow of qi and also has the function of ensuring free qi circulation. Since these characteristics are similar to the properties of wood, the liver is categorized as wood in the scheme of the five elements. Heart yang has a warming action so it belongs to the category of the fire element. The spleen is the source of transformation of essential substances and is associated with the earth element's characteristics of growth and transformation. The lung has clearing and descending properties and is associated with the metal element's characteristics of clearing and astringency. The kidney has the function of controlling water metabolism and storing essence and is associated with the water element's characteristics of moistening and flowing downward.

Copyright 2005 Hopkins Technology.

Our emotions are *interactive* in two ways, they interact with each other and they interact with the environment, with other people's emotions and even with surrounding natural energies such as the weather. Yes, our emotions influence the weather; this is not a superstition but one of the findings that Wilhelm Reich's *orgone research* has corroborated. *Vice versa*, the macrocosmic energies contained in the earth atmosphere, and even solar spots influence our emotions. There is nothing really separated in nature. All of us know the disastrous influence negative people can have over even a mass audience.

HOMEOPATHY

From Paracelsus to Masaru Emoto

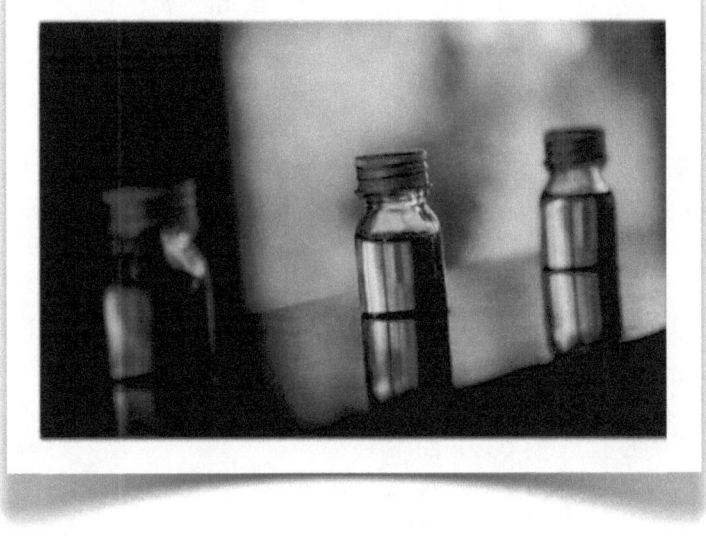

Introduction and References

In the following sub-chapters about Paracelsus, Samuel Hahnemann, Edward Bach and Masaru Emoto, I shall explain in detail how I came to try and use homeopathy and how wonderfully it helped to cure an almost fatal disease that was brought about by a continuous and irresponsible medical prescription of antibiotics against recurring diarrhea.

The most important general principle of homeopathy is that it restores the natural *yin-yang* balance in the organism by restoring the vital energy flow, and it does this by etheric substances that are dissolved in water, thereby using the *hado*, the memory of water, to hold on to the specific vibrations and transmit them to the client who drinks the water.

I would like to recommend to the reader the following publications, all of which I have not only studied but also reviewed in my *110 Book Reviews (2010)*.

Donna Eden

Energy Medicine (1999)
The Energy Medicine Kit (2004)
Energy Psychology (2005)

Masaru Emoto

The Hidden Messages in Water (2004)
The Secret Life of Water (2005)

Richard Gerber

A Guide to Vibrational Medicine (2001)

Shafica Karagulla

The Chakras (1989)

Ervin Laszlo

Science and the Akashic Field (2004)

Lynne McTaggart

The Field (2002)

Paracelsus

I read *Paracelsus (1493-1541)*, whose real name was *Theophrastus Philippus Aureolus Bombastus von Hohenheim* rather early in life, at the time when I was reading Franz Anton Mesmer, back in 1975, when I entered law school at age twenty. And I saw the similarity between the two otherwise very different personalities, regarding their discovery of the bioplasmatic energy, or *human energy field*.

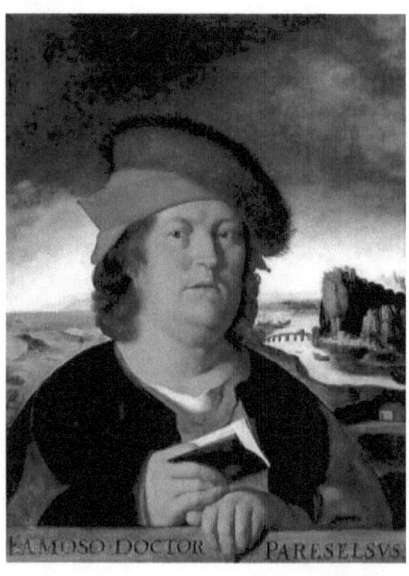

Paracelsus truly was a holistic healer. He continued an ancient tradition that for the majority in his time was completely lost. It was the *Hermetic Healing Tradition*. It must be noted that the breakup with this holistic healing tradition occurred not after the downfall of the Greek Empire, but in the midst of it. It was *Hippocrates*, who is often cited as the great medical benefactor of humanity, was actually the greatest detractor of true healing. Manly P. Hall writes in *The Secret Teachings of All Ages (2003)* about Hippocrates that he was the one single physician who, during the fifth century before Christ dissociated the healing arts from the other sciences of the temple and thereby established a precedent of separateness. Hall pursues:

Manly P. Hall

One of the consequences is the present widespread crass scientific materialism. The ancients realized the interdependence of the sciences. The moderns do not; and as a result, incomplete systems of learning are attempting to maintain isolated individualism. The obstacles which confront present-day scientific research are largely the result of prejudicial limitations imposed by those who are unwilling to accept that which transcends the concrete perceptions of the five primary human senses.[1]

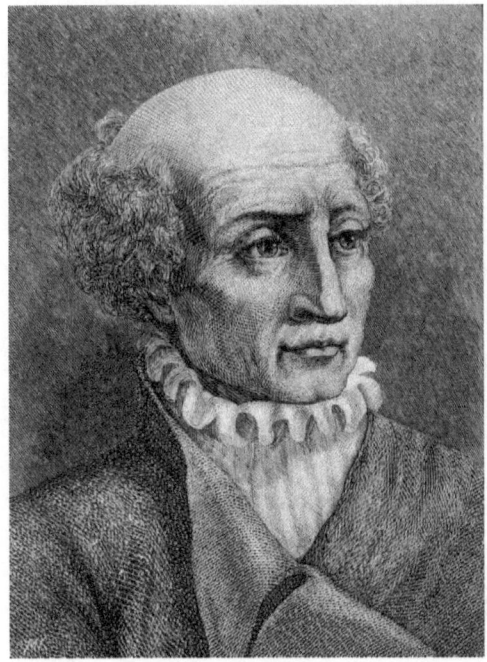

---

[1] Manly P. Hall, *The Secret Teachings of All Ages (2003)*, p. 344.

Below I will provide some more details about this tradition and how Paracelsus applied it in his own holistic approach to healing. But I would like to begin with the beginning, the starting principle of life as it were, that after all was never ever recognized in the West as a scientifically provable principle or pattern in both the macro – and the microcosm.

This principle or pattern is the *human energy field*, or cosmic life energy. Paracelsus discovered this force everywhere, and both in the plant and animal realm, and he called it *mumia* or *vis vitalis*. This is interesting because Mesmer who rediscovered this energy later, never bothered about plants and thought the energy was contained only in animals and humans.

Paracelsus, probably because he had understood that life is energy, and that all our dysfunctions in the body, as Chinese medicine knows since millennia, are obstructions of the vital energy flow, or *emotional flow*, was a phenomenally successful healer.[2] Yet because of his tempestuous character and his pride, he had to struggle hard against jealousy and also against the Church-driven authorities who reproached him he was doing black magic.

He had to stand trial for this cause, but he won the trial and was released. The social reject that was going along with his persecution was not too hard for him to bear as he was a *wandering scholar* and healer for long periods in his life, thus traveling around.

---

[2] See Pierre F. Walter, *Emotional Flow, Audio Book, 2010*.

From this knowledge that is to be found also in Chinese plant medicine, he lectured that certain plants are collateral for healing and certain others not. He proposed to take only the *essences* from these plants, as this was later done by Samuel Hahnemann and Edward Bach in homeopathy, and to distill them as tinctures in which their energetic

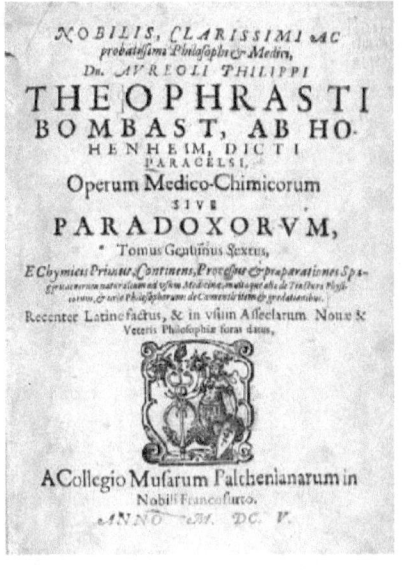

codes harmoniously melt into a higher form of unison vibration.

Here are some quotes from Manly P. Hall's book *The Secret Teachings of All Ages (2003)* about Paracelsus that I find so pertinent that I would like to reproduce them here. In chapter XXIV, and the first sub-chapter, entitled *The Paracelsian System of Medical Philosophy*, Manly P. Hall writes:

Manly P. Hall

Paracelsus felt that the healing of the sick was of far greater importance than the maintaining of an orthodox medical standing, so he sacrificed what might otherwise have been a dignified medical career and at the cost of lifelong persecution bitterly attacked the therapeutic systems of his day. He was a true explorer of Nature's arcanum. Many authorities have held the opinion that he was the discoverer of mesmerism, and that Mesmer evolved the art as the result of studying the writings of this great Swiss physician. The utter contempt which Paracelsus felt for the narrow systems of medicine in vogue during his lifetime, and his conviction of their inadequacy, are best expressed in his own quaint way: 'But the number of diseases that originate from some unknown causes are far greater than those that come from mechanical causes, and for such diseases our physicians know no cure because not knowing such causes they cannot remove them'.[3]

There is one vital substance in nature upon which all things subsist. It is called archaeus, or vital life force, and is synonymous with the astral light or spiritual air of the ancients. This vital energy has its origin in the spiritual body of the earth. Every created thing has two bodies, one visible and substantial, the other invisible and transcendent. The latter consists of an ethereal counterpart of the physical form; it constitutes the vehicle of archaeus, and may be called the vital body. This etheric shadow sheath is not dissipated by death, but remains until the physical form is entirely disintegrated. It is derangements of this astral light body that cause much disease.[4]

Paracelsus, recognizing derangements of the etheric double as the most important cause of disease, sought to reharmonize its substances by bringing into contact with it other bodies whose vital energy could supply elements needed, or were strong enough to overcome the diseased conditions existing in the aura of the sufferer. Its invisible cause having been thus removed, the ailment speedily vanished. The vehicle for the archaeus, or vital life force, Paracelsus called the mumia. A good example of a physical mumia is vaccine, which is the vehicle of a semi-astral virus. Anything which serves as a medium for the transmission of the archaeus, whether it be organic or inorganic, truly physical or partly spiritualized, was termed a mumia. The most universal form of mumia was ether, which modern science has accepted as a hypothetical sub-

---

[3] Id., p. 345.

[4] Id., p. 346.

stance serving as a medium between the realm of vital energy and that of organic and inorganic substance.[5]

Paracelsus discovered that in many cases plants revealed by their shape the particular organs of the human body which they served most effectively. The medical system of Paracelsus was based on the theory that by removing the diseased etheric mumia from the organism of the patient and causing it to be accepted into the nature of some distant and disinterested thing of comparatively little value, it was possible to divert from the patient the flow of the archaeus which had been continually revitalizing and nourishing the malady. Its vehicle of expression being transplanted, the archaeus necessarily accompanied its mumia, and the patient recovered.[6]

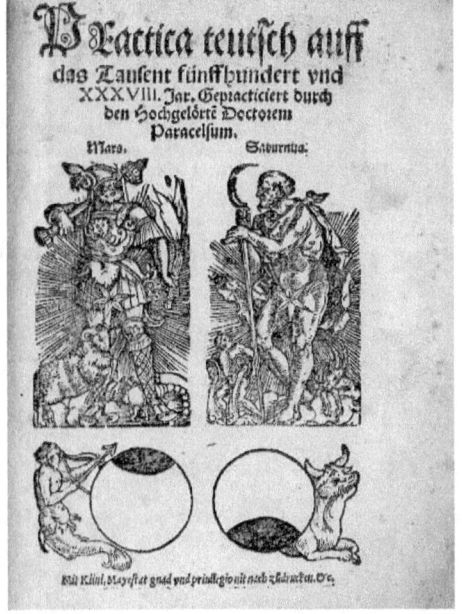

---

[5] Id., p. 347.

[6] Id.

Paracelsus' oeuvre is prolific both in quantity of content and scientific penetration. There are more than two hundred volumes of his writings still preserved, some hundred eighty of which are separately published editions before 1800.

This remarkable collection appears to have been amassed carefully over a period of twenty or so years, commencing with Ferguson's first essay in Paracelsian research; a paper to the University Dialectic Society in 1873, entitled simply, *Paracelsus*, and culminating in the purchase of the extensive *Paralcelsia* belonging to Dr. Eduard Schubert sometime in 1894.

Schubert, with his friend Karl Sudhoff, had been interested in Paracelsus since his student days, and together they published *Paracelsus-Forschungen* between 1887 and 1889. They had also collaborated on a comprehensive bibliography of Paracelsus editions.

This was subsequently completed by Sudhoff, and finally published in 1894, two years after Schubert's death at the age of seventy. In the introduction to his *Bibliographia Paracelsia* Sudhoff lists the numerous libraries that he has used in the compilation of this monumental work.

Samuel Hahnemann

I find it amazing how Hahnemann discovered the basic principles of homeopathy he, a traditional physician with an antipathy against medicine because, just like Paracelsus before him, who was appalled because of the blunt ignorance of Western medicine and the subtle and sometimes brutal treatments it bestowed upon the patient as the suffering agent. And just like Paracelsus, Hahnemann became aware

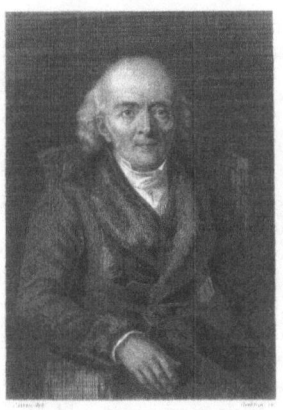

SAMUEL HAHNEMANN.

that traditional medicine was just treating the symptoms of diseases and had no idea of the underlying causes because it ignored a holistic and comprehensive concept of *health*.

Hahnemann began to systematically test substances for the effect they produced on a healthy individual and tried to deduce from this the ills they would heal. And he discovered that these dilutions, when done according to his technique of *succussion*, that is the systematic mixing through vigorous shaking, and *potentization*, were effective in producing symptoms. Thus, instead of directly jumping to curing symptoms, he was first producing those symptoms with substances – and the surprising discovery he made was that typically the substance that was producing the symptom was the one that was curing the disease.

Hahnemann began practicing medicine again using his new technique, which soon attracted other doctors. He first published an article about the homeopathic approach to medicine in a German medical journal in 1796; in 1810, he wrote his *Organon of the Medical Art*, the first systematic treatise on the subject. Let me give you a preview of this oeuvre, which is published entirely on the Internet.

Samuel Hahnemann

§1 The physician's high and only mission is to restore the sick to health, to cure, as it is termed. His mission is not, however, to construct so-called systems, by interweaving empty speculations and hypotheses concerning the internal essential nature of the vital processes and the mode in which diseases originate in the interior of the organism, (whereon so many physicians have hitherto ambitiously wasted their talents and their time); nor is it to attempt to give countless explanations regarding the phenomena in diseases and their proximate cause (which must ever remain concealed), wrapped in unintelligible words and an inflated abstract mode of expression, which should sound very learned in order to astonish the ignorant - whilst sick humanity sighs in vain for aid. Of such learned reveries (to which the name of theoretic medicine is given, and for which special professorships are instituted) we have had quite enough, and it is now high time that all who call themselves physicians should at length cease to deceive suffering mankind with mere talk, and begin now, instead, for once to act, that is, really to help and to cure.

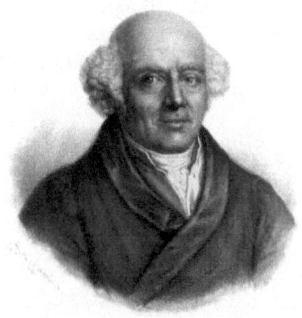

§2 The highest ideal of cure is rapid, gentle and permanent restoration of the health, or removal and annihilation of the disease in its whole extent, in the shortest, most reliable, and most harmless way, on easily comprehensible principles.

§3 If the physician clearly perceives what is to be cured in diseases, that is to say, in every individual case of disease (knowledge of disease, indication), if he clearly perceives what is curative in medicines, that is to say, in each individual medicine (knowledge of medical powers), and if he knows how to adapt, according to clearly defined principles, what is curative in medicines to what he has discovered to be undoubtedly morbid in the patient, so that the recovery must ensue - to adapt it, as well in respect to the suitability of the medicine most appropriate according to its mode of action to the case before him (choice of the remedy, the medicine indicated), as also in respect to the exact mode of preparation and quantity of it required (proper dose), and the proper period for repeating the dose; - if, finally, he knows the obstacles to recovery in each case and is aware how to remove them, so that the restoration may be permanent, then he understands how to treat judiciously and rationally, and he is a true practitioner of the healing art.

§4 He is likewise a preserver of health if he knows the things that derange health and cause disease, and how to remove them from persons in health.

§5 Useful to the physician in assisting him to cure are the particulars of the most probable exciting cause of the acute disease, as also the most significant points in the whole history of the chronic disease, to enable him to discover its fundamental cause, which is generally due to a chronic miasm. In these investigations, the ascertainable physical constitution of the patient (especially when the disease is chronic), his moral and intellectual character, his occupation, mode of living and habits, his social and domestic relations, his age, sexual function, etc., are to be taken into consideration.

§6 The unprejudiced observer - well aware of the futility of transcendental speculations which can receive no confirmation from experience - be his powers of penetration ever so great, takes note of nothing in every individual disease, except the changes in the health of the body and of the mind (morbid phenomena, accidents, symptoms) which can be perceived externally by means of the senses; that is to say, he notices only the deviations from the former healthy state of the now diseased individual, which are felt by the patient himself, remarked by those around him and observed by the physician. All these perceptible signs represent the disease in its whole extent, that is, together they form the true and only conceivable portrait of the disease.

Edward Bach

Introduction

Dr. Edward Bach (1886-1936) has contributed in a unique and outstanding way to homeopathy and generally, to natural healing. I came in touch with his flower remedies in 1997 when, returning from a two-year business trip from Asia to Germany, I was facing a dangerously low condition of vital energy due to a prolonged intake of antibiotics given from traditional doctors in order to fight recurring diarrhea.

From the natural healer I went to see, I learnt that the *therapeutic value* of Bach essences lies not in curing the physical symptoms of illness but in addressing the emotional state of the sufferer, wherein lie the roots of illness. For this reason the applica-

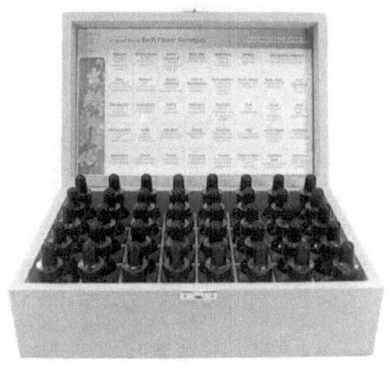

tion, I heard, of these 38 simple, natural essences spans the gamut, not only of human ailments, but also illnesses of other living beings. An emotional state, unlike an illness, crosses boundaries of species and illness type.

The most interesting in this kind of therapy was how the healer found the essence that was resonating with my illness. The female practitioner who had studied hypnosis and Reiki with a powerful Filipino healer, explained me very patiently the various methods for finding the energy essence corre-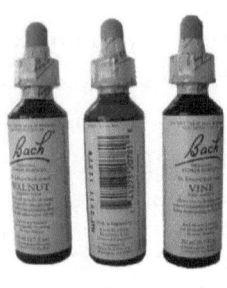sponding to my own organism's energy code and asked me which one I preferred. I chose the most direct method, hypnosis, and the experience was going to be a particularly revealing one for me. She was sitting at a forty-five degree angle at my right and asked me to put my left hand in her right hand. Then she told me to look in her eyes while she would take one flacon after the other in her left hand to sense the effect the vibration of the plant essence had on my organism.

Never before was I hypnotized so easily, so effectively and so joyfully. It was a very agreeable condition and I felt very clearly how each of the essences impacted energetically upon me.

The healer said I was going to feel either joyful, peaceful, positive and happy, which indicated that the essence was right for me, or I was feeling queer, anxious and negative, which was indicating that the essence was not compatible with my aura's vibrational structure. This was how I was going to choose one of the plant remedies. The treatment was the most effective one can imagine. It was almost miraculous. I was completely cured within three months, and with only six sessions.

By the time he died in 1936, Dr. Bach had discovered the 38 remedies that were needed to treat every possible emotional state, with each individual remedy being aimed at a particular emotion or characteristic. Sometimes people find it strange that only 38 can deal with everything, but in fact used in combination, over 292 million different mental states are covered.

Within the Bach flower system, and among the 38 essences, there are twelve plants that Bach himself called *The Twelve Healers*, which are of particular importance. I will briefly mention them below and describe them one by one.

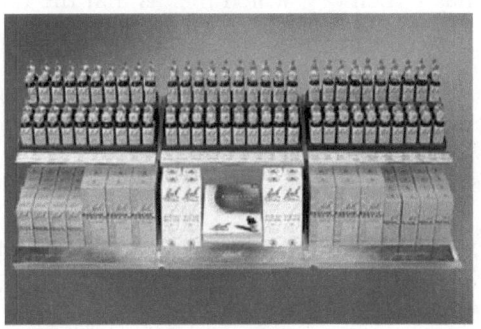

What Do Bach Flowers Do?

It is all about vibration we are talking when we talk about flower remedies. The universe is a vibrational cosmos with no finite particles, but dynamic energy patterns. Every flower has a unique energy pattern. There are energy frequencies that are particular to Agrimony, for example, and other energy frequencies that are characteristic for Gentian.

While perennial science since millennia understood that life is basically vibration, this is a relatively new insight for Western science, and it is now first of all quantum physics, and second, systems theory that brings the evidence long needed to integrated vibrational healing into the Western medical system.[7]

Water research has shown that flowers can cause water to vibrate with a different sort of energy. This means that the essence of the flower has a vibration that is imprinted upon the water in which it is placed. The water, being made up of vibrational energy itself, retains some of the vibration of the flower that was soaked in it. Masaru Emoto claims that water has a memory, which means that the flower's etheric imprint is stored in the water, and can actually be transferred from the water at a later time to other objects (or beings) also made of vibrational energy.

My research on emotions showed that all emotions have a particular energy – love, despair, anger, fear, revolt – one can consider each of these as a different vibrational pattern. Dr. Bach considered negative energetic states, negative emo-

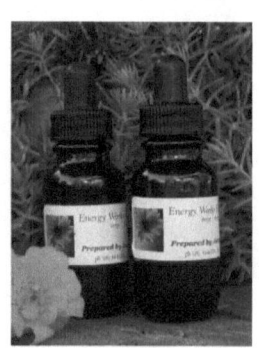

tions, to be the source of disease in the body, a theory supported by other natural healers. Dr. Bach also thought that these energetic states can be transformed, and that one of the transformational methods he discovered was the use of the *vibrational patterns* of flowers – it was then that *Flower Essence Therapy* was born.

Through basically a method of trial and error, Dr. Bach developed a system of therapy using the

[7] See Richard Gerber, *A Practical Guide to Vibrational Medicine (2001)*.

vibrational patterns of flowers, imprinted into spring water, to transform the emotional patters of human beings.

He showed through numerous case studies that plant essences, properly selected and applied, can be effective in treating the negative energies which underlie most disease states. Further, flower essences can be used to assist in transformation of any negative emotional state, be it temporary and transitive, or a more ingrained long-term pattern.

Dr. Bach's 12-7-19 Categorization Method

Dr. Bach categorized the original 38 flower essences he discovered into 3 categories to assist in their application. The categories are the *12 Healers* which reflect and transform our essential nature, the *7 Helpers* to assist with chronic conditions, and the *Second 19* that relate to more immediate traumas or difficulties. In the next paragraph, I shall describe the properties Dr. Bach assigned to each of these essences.

The Twelve Healers

The 12 Healers were designated by Dr. Bach as the flower essences that help the individual transform the source of discord at the very core of their being. These twelve essences are meant to address the twelve archetypal groups of humanity; the twelve primary personalities as Dr. Bach saw them. Some have gone so far as to relate these to the twelve signs of the Zodiac, though it is unclear as to whether this relationship was drawn by Dr. Bach himself. These twelve essences are an excellent starting point for any journey into flower essence healing, as it is often times our root disharmony or karmic imbalance that is the source of many ailments in our lives.

Agrimony

Dr. Bach

Are you one of those who suffer torments; who soul is restless: who can find no peace, and yet bravely face the world and hide your torture from your fellowmen: who laugh and smile and jest, and help those around you to keep a cheery

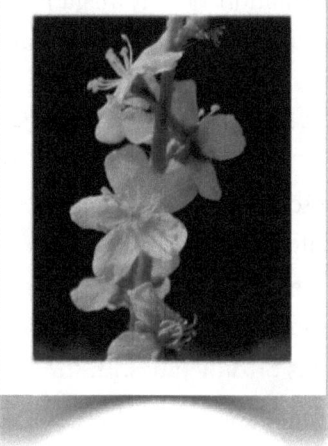

heart whilst you are suffering. Do you seek to soothe your sorrows by taking wine and drugs to help you face your trials: do you feel that you must have some stimulant in life to keep you going? If so, that beautiful plant Agrimony, growing along the sides of our lanes and in our meadows, with its church-like spire, and its seeds like bells, will bring you peace, the peace that 'passeth understanding'. The lesson of this plant is to enable you to hold peace in the presence of all trials and difficulties until no one has the power to cause you irritation. (Free Thyself, 1932)

Centaury

Dr. Bach

Are you one of those people whom everybody uses, because in the kindness of your heart you do not like to refuse them anything; do you just give in for the sake of peace rather than do what you know is right, because you do

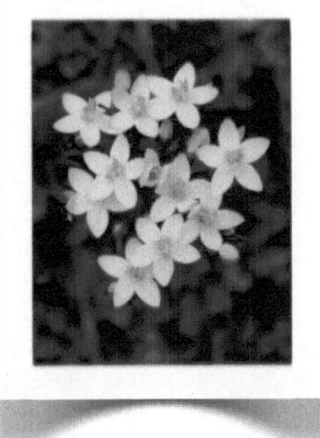

not wish to struggle; whose motive is good, but who are being passively used instead of actively choosing your own work? Those of you who are door-mats are a very long way along the road to being of great service once you can realise that you must be a little more positive in your life. Centaury, that grows in our pastures, will help you to find your real self, so that you may become an active, positive worker instead of a passive agent. (Free Thyself, 1932)

Cerato

Dr. Bach

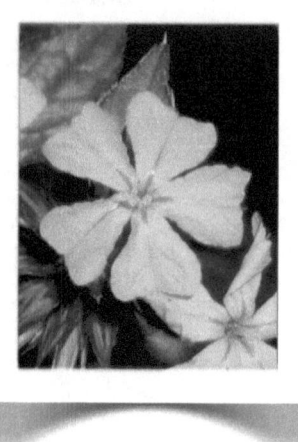

Are you one of those who feel that you have wisdom; that you could be a philosopher and a guide to your fellow-men? Do you feel the power within you to advise them in their difficulties, to soothe their sorrows, and at all times to be a help to them in their troubles; and yet, through lack of confidence in yourself, you are unable to accomplish this, possibly because you are listening too much to the voice of others and paying too great attention to the conventions of the world? Do you realise that it is only this lack of confidence in yourself, this ignorance of your own wisdom and knowledge, that tempts you to listen too intently to the advice of others? Then Cerato will help you to find your individuality, your personality, and, freed from outside influences, enable you to use the great gift of wisdom that you possess for the good of mankind. (Free Thyself, 1932)

Those who have not sufficient confidence in themselves to make their own decisions. They constantly seek advice from others, and are often misguided. (The 12 Healers and Other Remedies, 1936)

Chicory

Dr. Bach

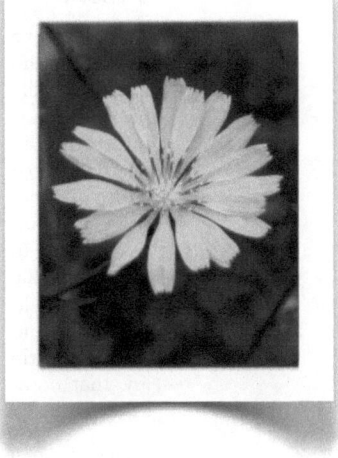

Are you one of those who long to serve the world, who long to open out both arms and bless all around you; who wish to help and comfort and sympathise, and yet for some reason circumstances or people stop you? Do you find that instead of serving many you are held in the grip of but a few, so that your opportunity of giving as fully as you wish is limited; are you getting to that stage when you wish to realise that it is, 'when all men count with you, but none too much?' Then that beautiful blue Chicory of the cornfields will help you to your freedom, the freedom so necessary to us all before we can serve the world. (Free Thyself, 1932)

Clematis

Dr. Bach

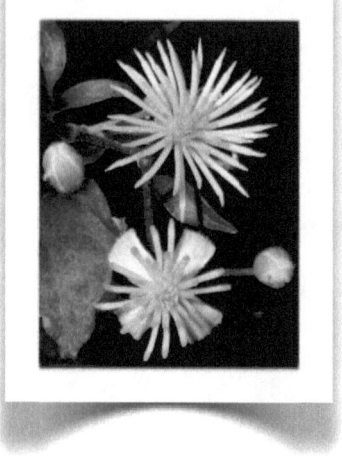

Are you one of those who find that life has not much interest, who wake almost wishing there were not another day to face, that life is so difficult, so hard, and has so little joy, that nothing really seems worth while, and how good it would be just to go to sleep, that it is scarcely worth the effort to try and get well? Have your eyes that far-away look as though you live in dreams and find the dreams so much more beautiful than life itself; or are your thoughts, perhaps, more often with someone who has passed out of this life? If you feel this way you are learning 'to hold on when there is nothing in you except the will which says to you - hold on!' and it is a very great victory to win through. (Free Thyself, 1932)

Those who are dreamy, drowsy, not fully awake, no great interest in life. Quiet people, not really happy in their present circumstances, living more in the future than in the present; living in hopes of happier times, when their ideals may come true. In illness some make little or no effort to get well, and in certain may even look forward to death, in the hope of better times; or maybe, meeting again some beloved one whom they have lost. (The 12 Healers and Other Remedies, 1936)

Gentian

Dr. Bach

Are you one of those with high ideals, with hopes of doing good; who find yourself dis- couraged when your ambitions are not quickly realised? When success is in your path are you elated, but when difficulties occur easily

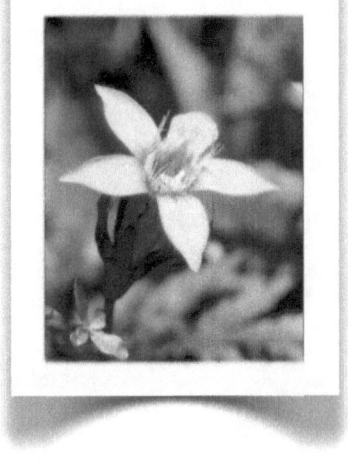

depressed? If so, the little Gentian of our hilly pastures will help you to keep your firmness of purpose, and a happier and more hopeful outlook even when the sky is over-cast. It will bring you encouragement at all times, and the understanding that there is no failure when you are doing your utmost, whatever the appar- ent result. (Free Thyself, 1932)

Those who are easily discouraged. They may be pro- gressing well in illness, or in the affairs of their daily life, but any small delay or hindrance to progress causes doubt and soon disheartens them. (The 12 Healers and Other Remedies, 1936)

Impatiens

Dr. Bach

Are you one of those who know that deep down in your nature there is still a trace of cruelty; when buffeted and harassed you find it difficult not to have a little malice? 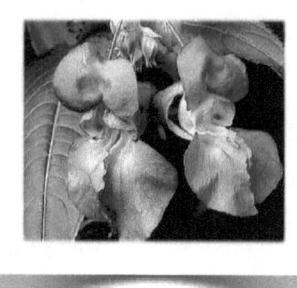 Have you still left within you the desire to use force to bring another to your way of thinking; are you impatient and does that impatience sometimes make you cruel; have you left in your nature any trace of the inquisitor? If so, you are striving for exquisite gentleness and forgiveness, and that beautiful mauve flower, Impatiens, which grows along the sides of some of the Welsh streams, will, with its blessing, help you along the road. (Free Thyself, 1932)

Mimulus

Dr. Bach

Are you one of those who are afraid; afraid of people or of circumstances, who go bravely on and yet your life is robbed of joy through fear, fear of those things that never happen, fear of people who really have no power over

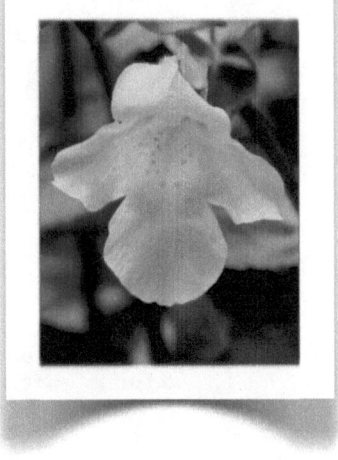

you, fear of tomorrow and what it may bring, fear of being ill or of losing friends, fear of convention, fear of a hundred things? Do you wish to make a stand for your freedom, and yet have not the courage to break away from your bonds; if so Mimulus, found growing on the sides of the crystal streams, will set you free to love your life, and teach you to have the tenderest sympathy for others. (Free Thyself, 1932)

Rock Rose

Dr. Bach

Are you one of those in absolute despair, in terror, who feel that you can bear nothing more; terrified as to what will happen, of death, of suicide, of insanity, of some awful disease; or fearful of facing the hopelessness of 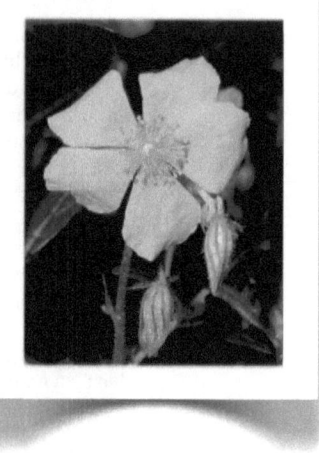 material circumstances? If so, you are learning to be brave against great odds, and fighting for your freedom, and the beautiful little yellow Rock Rose, which grows so abundantly on our hilly pastures, will give you the courage to win through. (Free Thyself, 1932)

Scleranthus

Dr. Bach

Are you one of those who find it difficult to make decisions; to form opinions when conflicting thoughts enter your mind so that it is hard to decide on the right course; when indecision dogs your path and delays your progress, does first

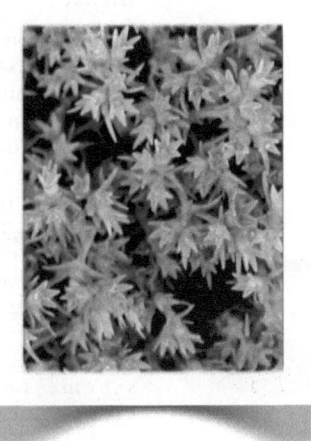

one thing seem right and then another? If so you are learning prompt action under trying circumstances; to form correct opinions and be steadfast in following them; and the little green Scleranthus of the cornfields will help you to this end. (Free Thyself, 1932)

Those who suffer much from being unable to decide between two things, first one seeming right then the other. They are usually quiet people, and bear their difficulty alone, as they are not inclined to discuss it with others. Those who have not sufficient confidence in themselves to make their own decisions. They constantly seek advice from others, and are often misguided. (The 12 Healers and Other Remedies, 1936)

Vervain

Dr. Bach

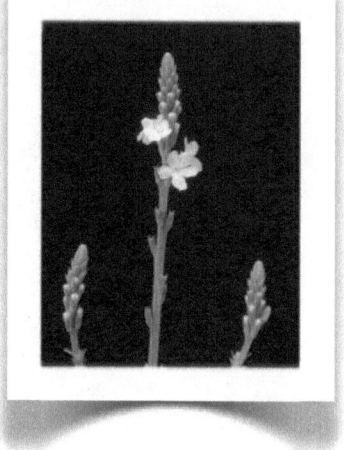

Are you one of those burning with enthusiasm: longing to do big things, and wishing all done in a moment of time? Do you find it difficult patiently to work out your scheme because you want the result as soon as you start? Do you find your very enthusiasm making you strict with others; wishing them to see things as you see them; trying to force them to your own opinions, and being impatient when they do not follow? If so, you have within you the power of being a leader and a teacher of men. Vervain, the little mauve flower of the hedge-banks, will help you to the qualities you need, kindness for your brothers, and tolerance for the opinions of others; it will help you to realise that the big things of life are done gently and quietly without strain or stress. (Free Thyself, 1932)

Water Violet

Dr. Bach

Are you one of those great souls who bravely and without complaint, still endeavouring to serve your brother-men, bear suffering calmly and with resignation, not allowing your grief to interfere with your daily work? Have you had 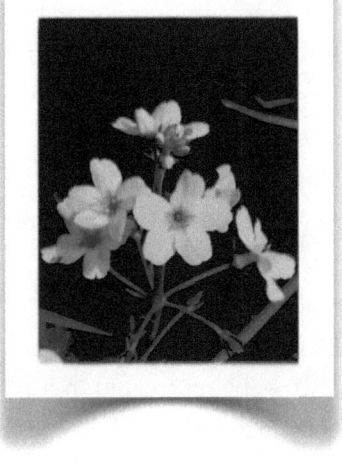 real losses, sad times, and yet go quietly on? (Free Thyself, 1932)

For those who in health or illness like to be alone. Very quiet people, who move about without noise, speak little, and then gently. Very independent, capable and self-reliant. Almost free of the opinions of others. They are aloof, leave people alone and go their own way. Often clever and talented. Their peace and calmness is a blessing to those around them. (The 12 Healers and Other Remedies, 1936)

Masaru Emoto

Dr. Masaru Emoto, Doctor of Alternative Medicine at the Open International University, Japan, and President of I.H.M. General Research Institute, became world-famous through the spectacular movie *'What the Bleep Do We Know'* *(2005)* and it was through this film that I got to know about his outstanding research on the memory of water.

When Dr. Emoto's books *The Hidden Messages in Water (2004)* and *The Secret Life of Water (2005)* reached me, they reached me right in time, at a moment when I had caught Dengue fever. But not only because was I in considerable distress being treated in a quite murky, unhealthy, inattentive and dirty Chinese hospital, the more significant thing about

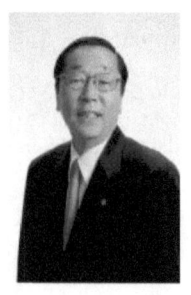

it is the date. The day the books arrived, was the 25th of July.

Dr. Emoto reports in *The Secret Life of Water* that according to the Mayan Calendar, the new year starts on July 26, and the day before was called 'the day out of time'. When you divide 365 by 28, you get 13 months and one extra day. This day was a celebration day during which prayers were offered.

And what I did that evening was to pray, with all my soul, and putting stickers with the words LOVE AND GRATITUDE on bottles with mineral water; in fact, I spent the whole evening reading *The Hidden Messages in Water*. As the serum treatment and injections I got in the hospital and the morning and the strong antibiotic pills I got for the afternoon rendered me very weak, tired, extremely sweaty and dizzy, I drank a lot of water and, following the advice of the doctor, was eating only rice porridge with fish. However, that evening was a silent prayer for the water inside of my body and indeed, the next morning I felt significantly better and for the first time, the fever was down.

That was the morning of the 26th of July. And for me it was indeed a new year. Dr. Emoto's voice, his *deep commitment* to the cause of a tortured earth, humankind and waters in distress has deeply penetrated into my soul and finds a complete resonance with the whole of my being. And the next day I composed 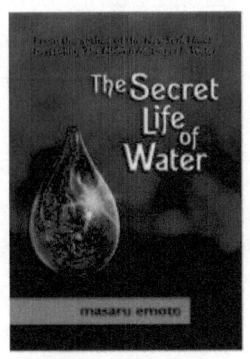 on the piano a little piece I entitled *Prayer to the Water*.

Without wanting to diminish Emoto's research in any way, I may want to mention that water research was not his invention. Max Freedom Long became aware that the Kahunas used a handy metaphor for describing the *mana* force; they associated it with water as a liquid substance that represents the juice of life; from this basic idea, the Kahunas extrapolated the metaphor of the human being as a tree or plant, 'the roots being the low self, the trunk and branches the middle self, and the leaves the high self'. While the sap circulating through roots, branches and leaves vividly illustrated the nature of the mana force.[8]

The *Essenes*, the first Christians gnostics, interestingly had the same or a very similar imagery regarding the vital force. It was for this reason, as Edmond Bordeaux-Szekely found, that they had given so much importance to the water purification ritual. They spoke of a *Goddess of the Water*, a 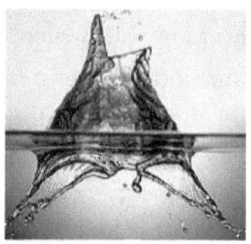 vital force that they believed was inhabiting water and that was purifying us through the use of daily cold showers taken in free nature and with water that was taken directly from a lively source such as a mountain stream or age-old well that was known to contain highly pure water.[9]

Now, the amazing research done with water and vibrations by Masaru Emoto fully confirms these findings with new and surprising evidence. Dr. Emoto found the enormous implications of vibration by looking at the vibrational code of water that he calls *hado*. In the Japanese spiritual tradition, *hado* is indeed considered as a vibrational code that, similar to *ki*, the life energy, has healing properties and transformative powers. Literally translated, *hado* means wave motion or vibration.

---

[8] See Max Long, The Secret Science at Work: The Huna Method as a Way of Life (1995), p. 17.

[9] See Edmond Bordeaux-Szekely, *Gospel of the Essenes (1988)*.

Once we are aware of it in our everyday lives, Emoto showed, *hado* can spark great changes in our physical space and emotional wellbeing. What Emoto teaches can thus be called hado awareness or *vibrational awareness*, as part of a general acute awareness of how we influence our environment, and our lives, through our thoughts and emotions. The point of departure is thus to recognize and acknowledge that in every thought and emotion, a specific vibration manifests.

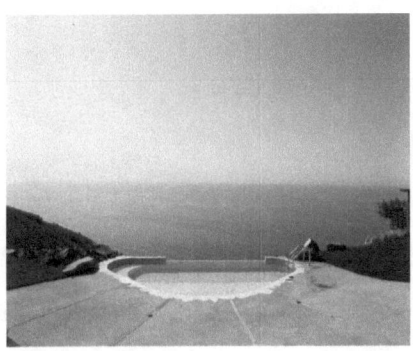

It is interesting that in *Feng Shui*, only flowing water is considered to contain the positive *ch'i* energy, while stagnant water is deemed to contain a rather harmful and retrograde variant of *ch'i* which is called *sha*.

The next amazing discovery that Emoto came about was the fact that water has a memory – a memory far longer than our transient lifetimes. And third, that we can learn from water, by allowing it to resonate within us. Only a few researchers have confirmed this assumption until now, and one of them is the reputed science philosopher Ervin Laszlo. Laszlo writes in his study *Science and the Akashic Field (2004)*:

Ervin Laszlo

Water has a remarkable capacity to register and conserve information, as indicated by, among other things, homeopathic remedies that remain effective even when not a single molecule of the original substance remains in a dilution.[10]

---

[10] Ervin Laszlo, *Science and the Akashic Field (2004)*, p. 53.

KIRLIAN PHOTOGRAPHY

The Final Evidence of the Luminous Energy Field

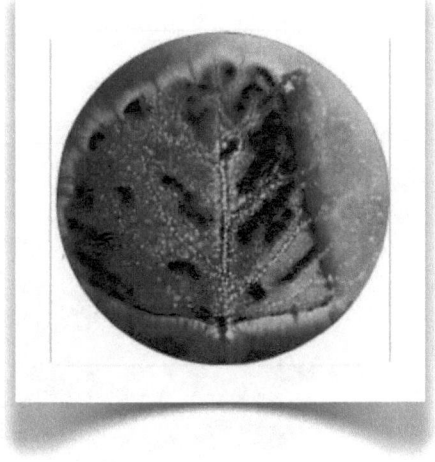

Kirlian Photography refers to a form of contact print photography, theoretically associated with high-voltage. It is named after Dr. Kirlian, who in 1939 discovered that if an object on a photographic plate is subjected to a strong electric field, an image is created on the plate. Dr. Kirlian's work, that was first called *corona discharge photography* was explored by other researchers such as Lichtenberg and Tesla. Yet Kirlian took the development of the effect further than any of his predecessors.

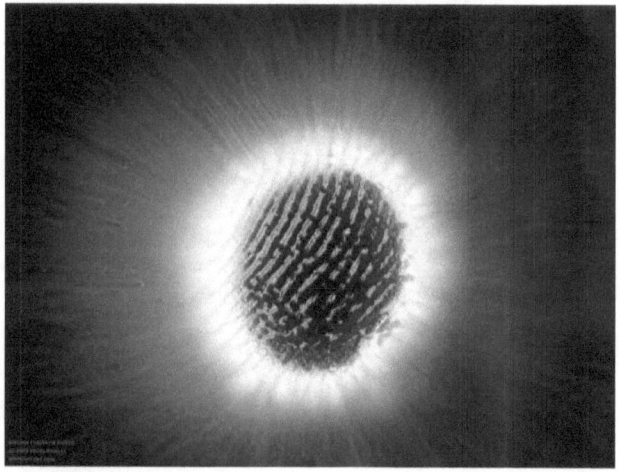

Kirlian Photography is today credited with being the first attempt to successfully photograph the bioplasmatic *aura* or *energy field* around living beings, plants, animals and humans. The photographs show the aura as a colorful halo stretching a few inches around the physical body.

One of the more striking aspects of Kirlian photography is its ability to illuminate the acupuncture points of the human body. An experiment advanced as *evidence of energy fields* generated by living entities involves taking Kirlian contact photographs of a picked leaf at set periods, its gradual withering being said to correspond with a decline in the strength of the aura.

Another striking fact proven by Kirlian photography is that the aura bears the memory of the whole body even when a part of the body is lost. This was shown with cutting off a leaf from a branch. The Kirlian photo still shows the missing leaf, which gave rise to explaining the fact why war veterans can indeed suffer from post-amputation pain in their missing arms or legs, a fact that previously was always downplayed as paranoid or a product of vivid fantasy.

It was back in the 1980s that I heard for the first time about Kirlian Photography for the first time. I thought for myself that that *had to be invented* as since my school days I had been aware that Western science is blinding out the most essential, the cosmic life energy, the bioplasmatic energy

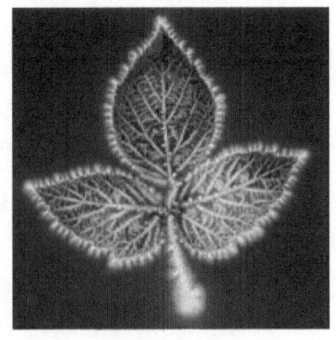

that is both in the cell plasma and the aura. Kirlian photography was perhaps the first convincing evidence of this energy.

I also became aware that with so many great discoveries, including *Reich's Greatest Discoveries*, which I describe in my audio book of the same title and in *The Science of Orgonomy*

(2010), they have been made in the first decades of the 20th century but were ferociously aggressed by the science establishment at first, and until today are more or less blinded out from the mainstream Western scientific worldview. Many of these discoveries have been promoted by those, who like Wilhelm Reich, were defamed and labeled as quacks and charlatans, but who, as we know today, were simply scientific geniuses.

It was at that time that I had my first ideas about creating a science that inquires into emotions and sexuality from the bioenergetic perspective and that I later called *Emonics*.[11] I was especially baffled by the fact that Kirlian Photography revealed the fact that memory is coded in the aura or the luminous body, which shows that *memory is actually a function of the luminous energy field*, not a matter of neurons and of mysterious substances in the brain.

Hence, memory is not located in the brain, and as this fact is in such flagrant contradiction with the myths of neurology and brain research, I was encouraged to research further on these lines.

There are several books among those I discussed in my book reviews that take reference to Kirlian Photography, one of them with more than a short reference. It is this book, which I highly recommend:

Shafica Karagulla

The Chakras
With Dora van Gelder Kunz

---

[11] See my audio book of the same title, published in 2010.

Correlations between Medical Science and Clairvoyant Observation (1989)

KYODO

A Japanese Martial Art

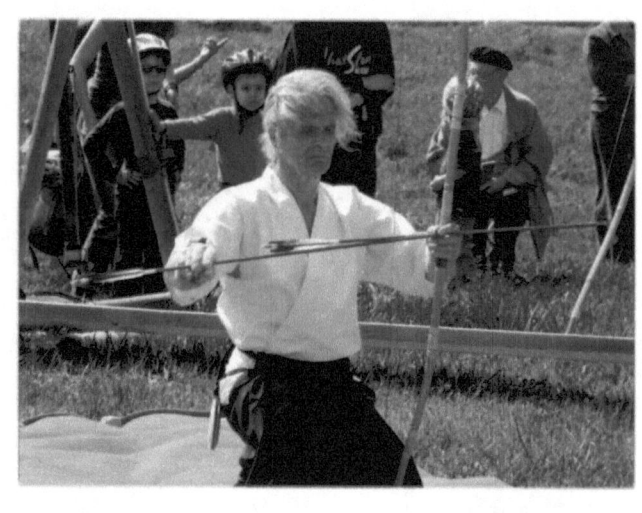

What is Kyodo

Kyudo, literally meaning way of the bow, is the Japanese art of archery. It is a modern Japanese martial art *(gendai budo)*. It is estimated that there are approximately half a million practitioners of Kyodo today.

In Japan, by most accounts, the number of female Kyodo practitioners is at least equal to or greater than the number of male practitioners. In its purest form, Kyodo is practiced as an art and as a means of moral and spiritual development.

Kyodo in Germany

Many archers practice Kyodo as a sport, with marksmanship being paramount. However, the goal most devotees of Kyodo seek is correct shooting and correct hitting. When the spirit and balance of the shooting is correct the result will be for the arrow to arrive in the target, which is of course a metaphor for success in life at large.

Kyodo in Japan

To give oneself completely to the shooting is the spiritual goal. In this respect, many Kyodo practitioners believe that competition, examination, and any opportunity that places the archer in this uncompromising situation is important, while other practitioners will avoid competitions or examinations of any kind.

NATUROPATHY

An American Natural Healing System

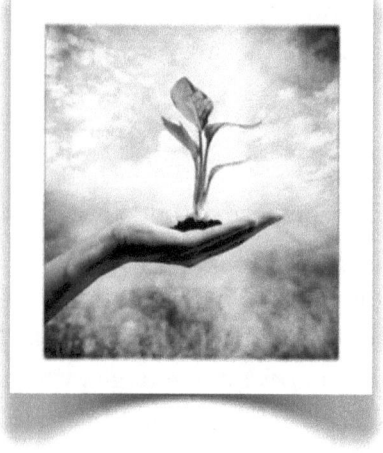

The Six Principles of Healing

1. Nature's Healing Power
2. Identify the Cause
3. Do No Harm
4. Whole Person Treatment
5. The Physician is Teacher
6. Disease Prevention

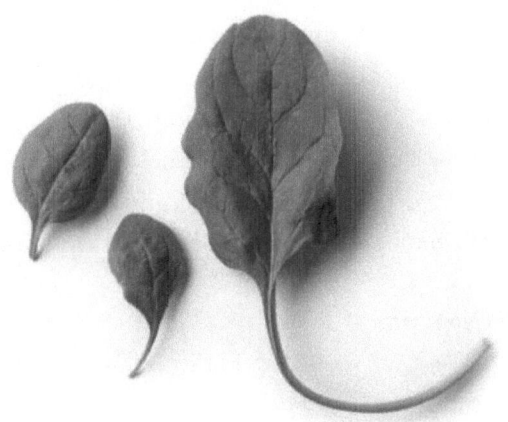

Nature's Healing Power

Using nature's inherent healing power implies to activate the body's self-healing ability, so that nature can exhibit its full healing power. Following this principle means the doctor should instruct the patient about getting enough sleep, doing some kind of exercise, feeding the body in natural ways and, if needed, considering a special diet, such as eating herbs, or algae, which as living organisms are antioxidants and contain the *essence of life.* Plants can gently move the body into health without side effects posed by some synthetic chemicals in modern pharmaceuticals.

Identify the Cause

We have seen that Samuel Hahnemann strongly emphasized to find the root cause of the disease instead of speculating what the various symptoms may do or not do to the body.

It is logical that for healing to occur, the root cause of the disease must be found and eliminated. The cause of the disease may be located at various levels at once, the physical, mental, emotional, and spiritual levels. It is the naturopathic doctor's ostensible role to identify this root cause, in addition to alleviating suffering by treating symptoms.

Do No Harm

We have seen that Paracelsus was strongly motivated to become a natural healer because he saw the great harm doctors did to their patients at that time. This principle is perhaps the most important for natural healing in general, and for naturopathy, in particular. It goes without saying that the treatment of the disease should never do greater harm than the disease itself.

Whole Person Treatment

It goes without saying that an approach that targets the root cause of the disease, instead of curing the symptoms, is one that approaches the whole human, and eventually heals the whole human – not just body parts. That means treating the entire body, as well as the spiritual being within the physical person.

The Physician is Teacher

It is the role of the natu-
ropath to educate the patient
in naturopathic practice and
encourage him or her to take
responsibility for their health
and wellbeing. This coopera-
tive relationship between doctor and patient is essential to

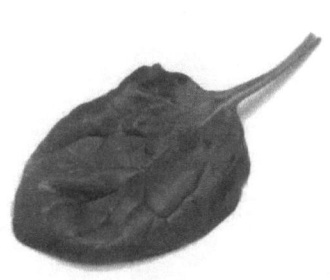

healing, while in modern medicine it is often neglected and replaced by applying machinery to the body 'machine' of the patient.

Disease Prevention

The ultimate goal of the naturopathic physician is prevention. The emphasis is on building health, not fighting illness. This is done by fostering healthy lifestyles, healthy beliefs, and healthy relationships.

OSTEOPATHY

The Eight Principles of Osteopathic Healing

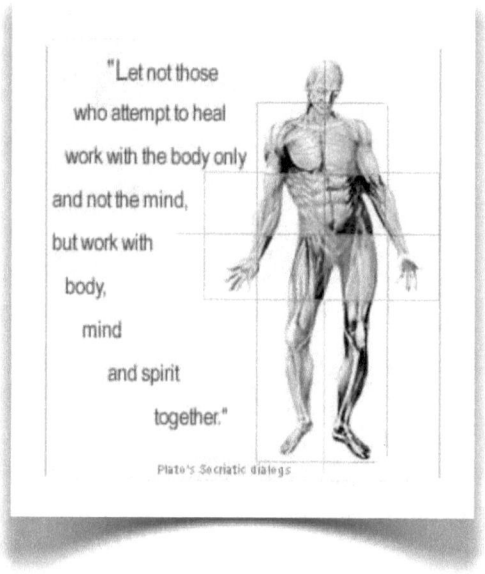

"Let not those who attempt to heal work with the body only and not the mind, but work with body, mind and spirit together."

Plato's Socratic dialogs

What is Osteopathy?

Osteopathy is a uniquely American natural health care system that was developed about one hundred twenty years ago.

With a strong emphasis on the inter-relationship of the body's nerves, muscles, bones and organs, osteopaths apply the philosophy of treating the whole person.

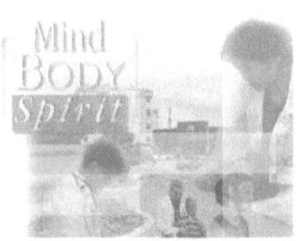

Osteopathy is thus a holistic approach to healing, which includes prevention, diagnosis and treatment of illness, disease and injury using manual and physical therapies (OMM).

For non-American natural healers it may be difficult to understand the difference between osteopathy and naturopathy. It has been for me.

Osteopathic medicine is practiced by osteopathic physicians in the United States. Osteopaths educated in countries outside the U.S. are referred to by American osteopathic physicians as 'non-physician osteopaths'. Their scope of practice is limited largely to musculoskeletal conditions and treatment of some other conditions using manual treatment (OMM), not unlike chiropractors (although the distinction between the two professions remains important to both).

The Eight Principles of Osteopathy

These are the eight major principles of osteopathy and are widely accepted throughout the osteopathic community.

They are taken from the curriculum of the *Kirksville College of Osteopathic Medicine:*

▸ (1) The body is a unit.

▸ (2) Structure and function are reciprocally inter-related.

▸ (3) The body possesses self-regulatory mechanisms.

▸ (4) The body has the inherent capacity to defend and repair itself.

▸ (5) When the normal adaptability is disrupted, or when environmental changes overcome the body's capacity for self maintenance, disease may ensue.

▸ (6) The movement of body fluids is essential to the maintenance of health.

▸ (7) The nerves play a crucial part in controlling the fluids of the body.

▸ (8) There are somatic components to disease that are not only manifestations of disease, but also are factors that contribute to the maintenance of the disease state.

These principles are not held by osteopaths to be empirical laws, nor contradictions to orthodox medical principles; they are thought to be the underpinnings of the osteopathic perspective on health and disease.

QIGONG

The Art of Breathing

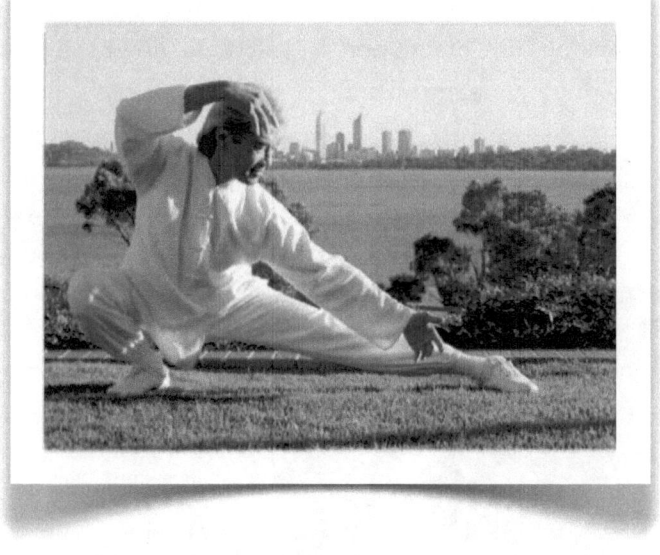

What is Qigong?

Qigong or *ch'i kung* refers to a wide variety of traditional cultivation practices that involve methods of accumulating, circulating, and working with the vital energy flow *(ch'i)* mainly through breathing and other body energy work.

Qigong is practiced for health maintenance purposes, as a therapeutic intervention, as a medical profession, a spiritual path and/or component of Chinese martial arts. The *ch'i* or *qi* means 'air' in Chinese, and, by extension, *life force*, dynamic energy or even cosmic breath.

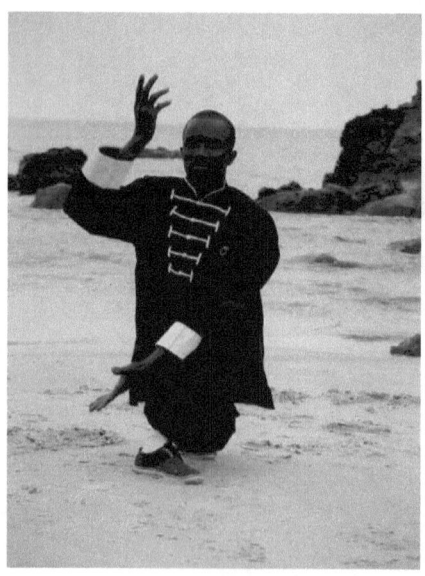

Gong means work applied to a discipline or the resultant level of skill; qigong is thus breath work or energy work.

Wikipedia

Most Western medical practitioners and many practitioners of traditional Chinese medicine, as well as the Chinese government, view qigong as a set of breathing and movement exercises, with possible benefits to health through stress reduction and exercise. Others see qigong in more metaphysical terms, claiming that qi can be circulated through channels called meridians.

The Qigong Posture

Qigong is a Chinese system of breath control and physical postures that support right breathing. Right breathing activates the flow of the *ch'i* or vital energy in the organism and thereby helps prevent disease. It also helps accelerating healing processes.

I have practiced Qigong over years and can testify that it purifies our inner energy channels, and contributes to health and mental clarity. It also helps to balance our emotions.

When practicing Qigong, one should ideally be on a healthy diet, avoid alcoholic beverages, avoid smoking and eat lots of fresh food, salads, sprouts, beans and fibers. One should also avoid dairy products.

Qigong for Healing Sadism

For people who suffer from a sadistic affliction, or recurrent strong rape desires, I recommend Qigong, among other self-awareness techniques, as I have elaborated them in various publications, among them my audio books *Emonics (2010), Emotional Flow (2010)*, as well as my *Idiot Guide to Love (2010)*.

Qigong clarifies and clears strayed energy patterns in our human aura, and brings them back into the unified energy field, so that sexual attraction is again tender, warm, with hot melting emotions and streaming sensations in the body, instead of the cold and violent urge for quick and sometimes brutal abreaction that characterizes the sadistic affliction.

RADIONICS

The Unknown Medical Science

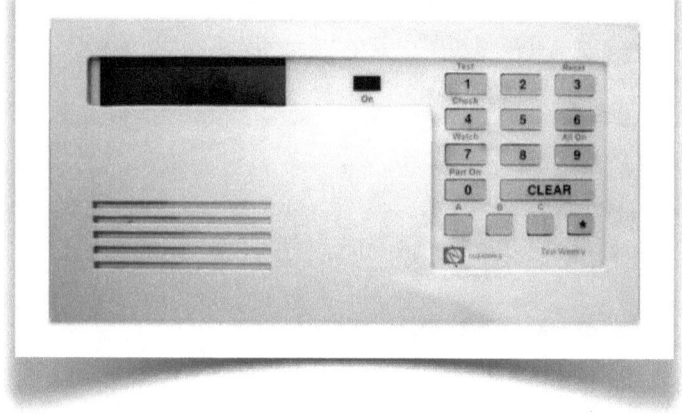

What is Radionics?

Radionics is a science that to this day is understood only by a small elite of scientists, as it is so far still largely located within the gray area between official science and spirituality, out of the shot lines of the great public.

But that does not diminish its importance. It owns its existence to two *rather distinct* streams of influence, for one the esoteric spiritual teachings of Alice Bailey, on one hand, and the experimental findings of the Russian-French scientist *Georges Lakhovsky (1869-1942)*, on the other. To explain the complex technique of this science in simple words, let me describe

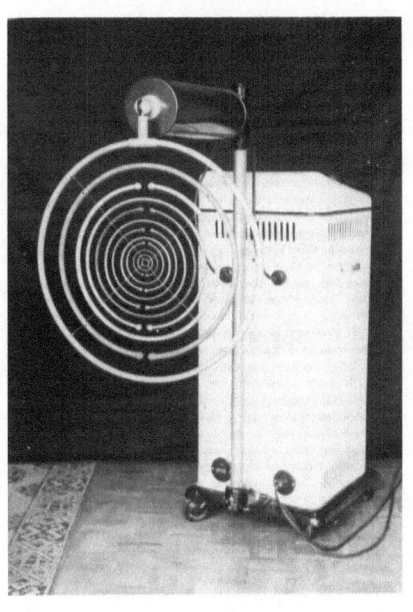

Radionics as a healing technique that uses insights into the laws of cell vibration for the purpose of healing illness.

Radionics has been compared with Wilhelm Reich's *orgonomy*, with the laying-on of hands and with spiritual healing, but matters are more complex than that.[12] An in-depth

---

[12] See Pierre F. Walter, *The Science of Orgonomy, Monograph (2010)*.

study of this complex science would be needed to really explain its functioning.

Further Information and References
David K. Tansley, *Chakras-Rays and Radionics (1984)*

The Pioneer

I have reviewed George Lakhovsky's major writings, among them *The Secret of Life (1929)* in my *110 Book Reviews (2010)*.

Lakhovsky found that all living cells possess attributes that normally are associated with electronic circuits. From this starting point and the observation that the oscillation of high frequency sine waves when sustained by a small, steady supply of outside energy of the right frequency would bring about what Lakhovsky called *resonance*, he conducted experiments showing that living cells respond to oscillations imposed upon them from outside sources. This outside source of radiation was attributed by Lakhovsky to cosmic rays that constantly bombard the earth. On the basis of these insights, Lakhovsky construed devices for healing by the application of high frequency waves, that today we know as *Radionics*.

Lakhovsky found that when outside sources of oscillations are resonating in synch with the energy code of the cell, the cell's growth would become stronger, while when frequencies differed, this would weaken the vitality of cell. From this primary observation, Lakhovsky further found that the cells of pathogenic organisms produce different frequencies than that of normal, healthy cells.

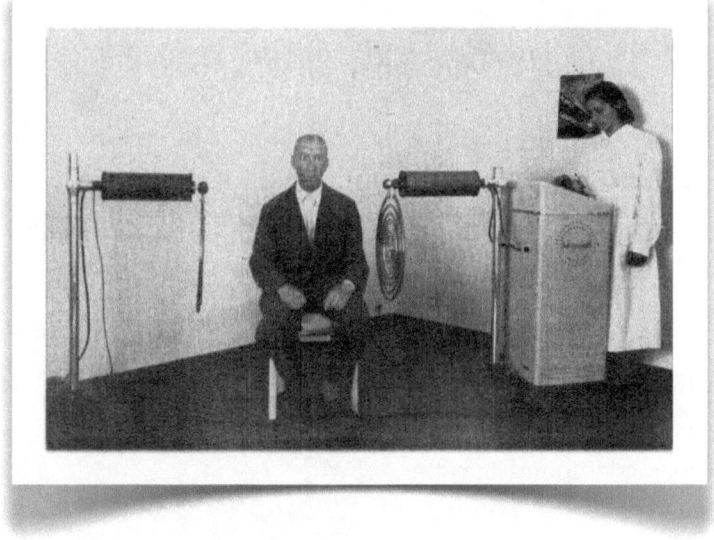

Lakhovsky specifically observed that if he could increase the amplitude, but not the frequency, of the oscillations of healthy cells, this increase would dampen the oscillations produced by disease-causing cells, thus bringing about their decline. However, when he rose the amplitude of the disease causing cells, their oscillations would gain the upper hand and cause the person or plant to become weaker and more ill.

As a result of these observations, Lakhovsky viewed the progression of disease as essentially a battle between resonant oscillations of host cells versus oscillations emanating from pathogenic organisms.

He initially proved his theory using plants. In December, 1924, he inoculated a set of ten germanium plants with a plant cancer that produced tumors. After thirty days, tumors had developed in all of the plants, upon which Lakhovsky took one of the ten infected plants and simply fashioned a heavy copper wire in a one loop, open-ended coil about thirty centimeter (12") in diameter around the center of the plant and held it in place. The copper coil was found to collect and concentrate energy from extremely high frequency cosmic rays.

The diameter of the copper loop determined which range of frequencies would be captured. Lakhovsky found that the *thirty centimeter loop* captured frequencies that fell within the resonant frequency range of the plant's cells. This captured energy thus reinforced the resonant oscillations naturally produced by the nucleus of the germanium's cells.

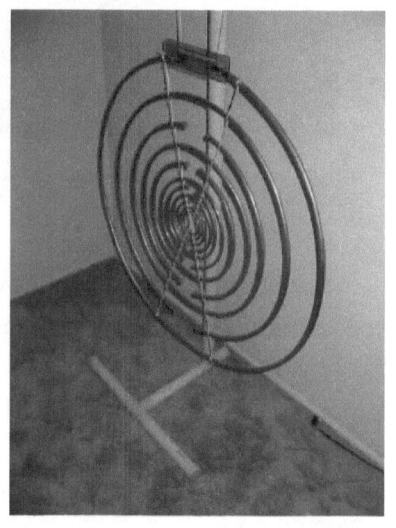

This allowed the plant to overwhelm the oscillations of the cancer cells and destroy the cancer. The tumors fell off in less than three weeks and by two months, the plant was thriving. All of the other cancer-inoculated plants, those that were not receiving the copper coil, died within thirty days.

Lakhovsky then fashioned loops of copper wire that could be worn around the waist, neck, elbows, wrists, knees, or ankles of people and found that over time relief of painful symptoms was obtained. These simple coils, worn continuously around certain parts of the body, would invigorate the vibrational strength of cells and increased the immune response which in turn took care of the offending pathogens.

Upon which Lakhovsky construed a device that produced a broad range of high frequency pulsed signals that radiate energy to the patient via two round resonators: one resonator acting as a transmitter and the other as a receiver. The machine generates a very wide spectrum of high frequencies coupled with static high voltage charges applied to the resonators. These high voltages cause a corona discharge around the perimeter of the outside resonator ring that Lakhovsky called *effluvia*. The patient sat on a wooden stool in between the two resonators and was exposed to these energies for about fifteen minutes. The frequency waves *sped up the recovery process* by stimulating the resonance of healthy cells in the patient and in doing so, increased the immune response to the disease organisms.

To summarize, all these researchers saw the interactive link or resonance between cell vibration, which I call *emonic vibration*, and health or disease.[13]

And all of them were able to construe devices or even work without devices to influence and manipulate cell vibration so as to strengthen immunitary response and fighting pathologies. The process was particularly evident in George Lakhovsky's research in that it was experimentally demon-

---

[13] See Pierre F. Walter, *Emonics, Audio Book (2010)*.

strated how a simple device, because it brought about a resonance with the cell's emonic vibration, could actively fight a
cancerous tumor in the plant and thus eliminate the cancer.

Lakhovsky called the cosmic energy *universion*, which is
the title of one of his lesser known books, published 1929 in
Paris, in French language. I have called this force *e-force*.[14]

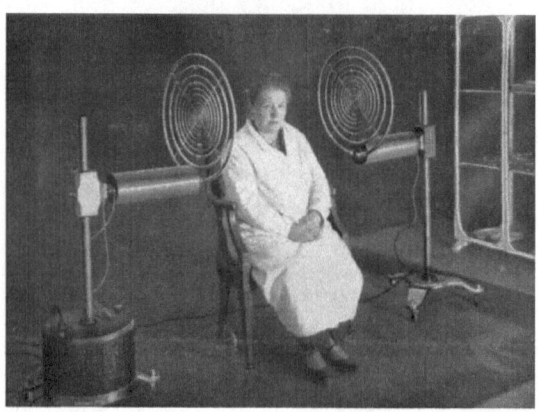

---

[14] See *Walter's Encyclopedia, Academic Edition (2010)*.

REIKI

The Usui System

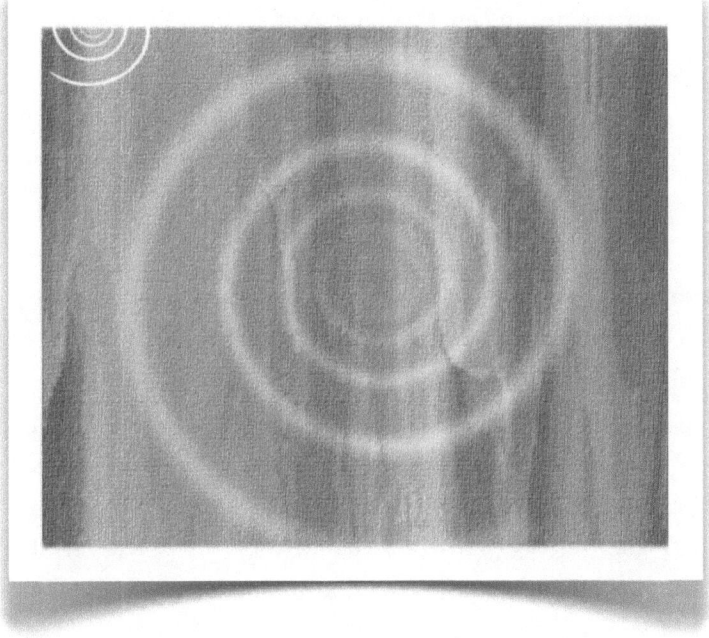

Reiki is a spiritual practice developed in 1922 by Mikao Usui. After three weeks of fasting and meditating on Mount Kurama, in Japan, Usui claimed to receive the ability of healing without energy depletion.

A portion of the practice, tenohira or palm healing, is used as a form of *complementary and alternative medicine (CAM)*. Tenohira is a technique whereby practitioners believe they are moving healing energy (a form of *ki*) through the palms.

Wikipedia

There is no generally accepted scientific evidence for either the existence of ki or any mechanism for its manipulation, and a systematic review of randomized clinical trials conducted in 2008 did not support the efficacy of reiki or its recommendation for use in the treatment of any condition.

The Wikipedia article shows the pitiful ignorance of not only our society as a whole, but the bunch of people signed up for this encyclopedia that seems to have been set out to preserve as much as possible not only the fundamental Cartesian blind-out of their founders, but of the whole of Cartesian fake science. How else could they be so successful, if they were not swimming on the mainstream of blind-and-deaf consumer stupidity?

Reiki is energy-based healing. It works with what the Japanese call *ki* and what I call *e-force*.[15] Variants of energy healing exist in virtually all cultures around the world, while I

---

[15] See, Pierre F. Walter, *Emonics, Audio Book (2010)* as well as *The Idiot Guide to Emotions (2010), The Idiot Guide to Science (2010)* and *The Idiot Guide to Soul Power (2010)*.

must say that the Japanese have a more direct connection to it still today because of the *Shinto* religion that is one of the few in the world, next to only *Huna*, that officially recognizes psychic powers, and the invisible world, as a scientific fact, not as in dominator religions, as a religious dogma that is hammered in the minds and hearts of their believers.

Mikao Usui has rediscovered the Reiki system at the beginning of the 20th century, while Reiki is something like a perennial natural healing technique and as such thousands of years old.

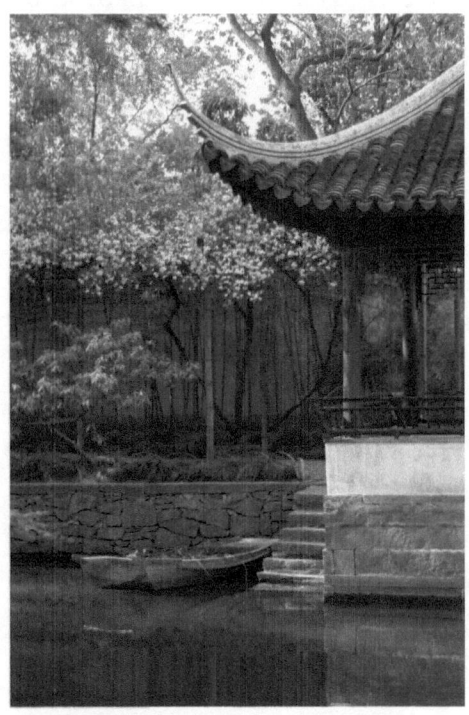

I came in touch with Reiki in 1994 through the friendship with Anneke van Gelder, a Reiki master practicing in Rotterdam, Holland, where I ran my own consulting company from 1994 to 1996, located in the *Beurs World Trade Center*. But my ideas were not really turning toward business, which is why I finally gave up that company and focused on my interests in healing and coaching people. With Anneke, then, I learnt Reiki, the whole of the theory and the practice, and to my astonishment she told me that my rei-ki (from Japanese: intelligent energy) energy was very high. So I accomplished the first degree in Reiki in that year.

SOPHROLOGY

The Study of the Harmony of Consciousness

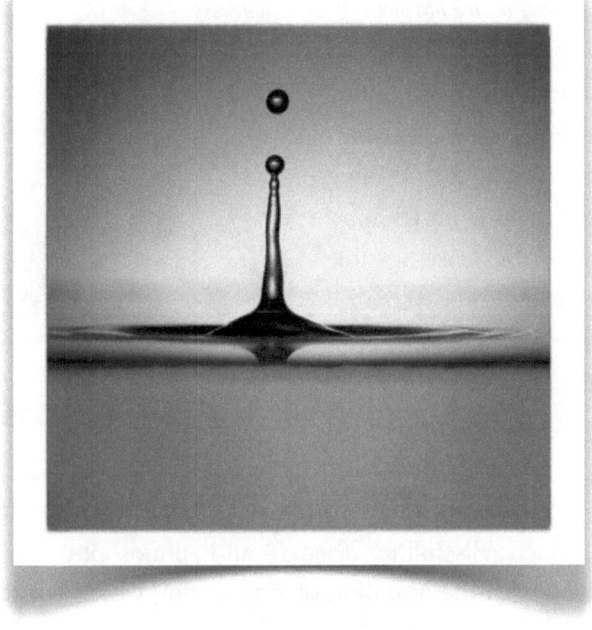

What is Sophrology?

Sophrology was created by Dr. Alfonso Caycedo in the 1960s. It is a branch of mindbody psychology that focuses on understanding human consciousness and altered states of consciousness for short-term or long-term positive modifications, relaxation and purposes of personal growth and creativity boosting. The term is derived from old Greek and means *study of the harmony of consciousness.*

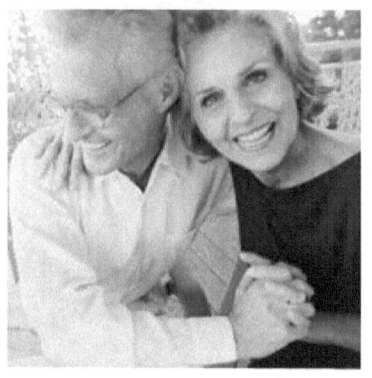

Caycedo originally set out to find a way of healing depressed and trauma-ridden clients by leading them to health and happiness with the least possible use of drugs and psychiatric treatments. He journeyed extensively to study the Eastern philosophies of Yoga, Zen and Buddhism, each time viewing them within a Western scientific framework. Each discipline, theory and philosophy was approached with the intention of discovering what, exactly, improved people's health, both physically and mentally, in the fastest possible time and with lasting results.

On his return Professor Caycedo designed a method of healing, creating a 12 level training program from both Eastern and Western philosophies that took into account our modern way of life – with its speed, stress and problems. The training is divided into 3 cycles – the *reduction cycle*, the *radical cycle* and the *existential cycle*. Professor Caycedo named his method *Sophrology* in 1960 and called it 'a training of the consciousness and the values of existence,' or 'Health & Happiness Training'. Now, after 45 years of research, fine tuning and experimentation, he has extensive evidence of the effectiveness of the Sophrology method.

Sophrology is a structured method created to produce optimal health and wellbeing. It consists of a series of easy -to-do physical and mental exercises that, with regular practice, lead to a healthy, relaxed body and a calm, alert mind. The exercises are called *dynamic relaxation (relaxation in movement)*.

The first things people generally notice are a more restful sleep, improved concentration, fewer worries, increased self-confidence, and a feeling of inner happiness.

Statistics

Athletes coached by Dr Raymond Abrezol between 1964 and 2004 have won over 200 Olympic medals. Generally speaking, sophrology is much more common in French-speaking countries than in the Anglo-Saxon world. Here are some statistics that show it.

Over 300,000 members of the public have followed courses of sophrology in French-speaking Switzerland over the last 25 years. Over three thousand medical, social and pedagogical professionals have followed the train-the-trainers lessons.

Sophrology was initially firmly within the field of psychiatry and medicine until Dr Raymond Abrezol discovered its unique benefits, and brought it to the attention of the great public. After practicing Sophrology for a while, Dr Abrezol began to observe a noticeable improvement in his tennis game. As an experiment, he introduced his opponents to the method, and they began to see their tennis vastly improve. He was consequently invited to coach the Swiss ski team and other Olympic athletes.

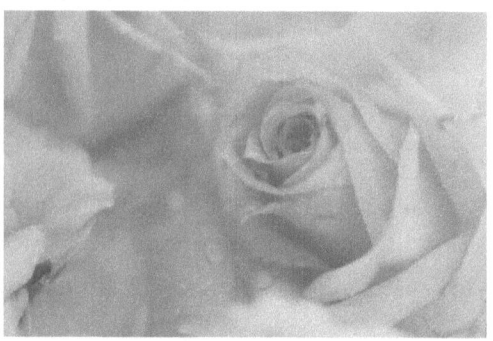

Growth in the French-Speaking World

The rapid growth of Sophrology throughout the French-speaking world can largely be attributed to Dr Abrezol running trainer training programs for a large number of influential doctors and sports coaches, many of whom now run centers throughout France. His enthusiasm and his success with athletes opened doors for Sophrology to be taught in many areas of life.

Benefits

Sophrology assists to rediscover our self-confidence and hidden potential. Group classes bring improvements in communications and interpersonal relations. Students have a stronger resistance to stressful situations, whether mental or physical. Since they have many more choices of how to act and react, it is easier to break out of old habitual patterns into more successful ways of operating.

The most important part is regular practice until the benefits of the Sophrology Training become part of every-day life.

TAI CHI CHUAN

The Soft Martial Art

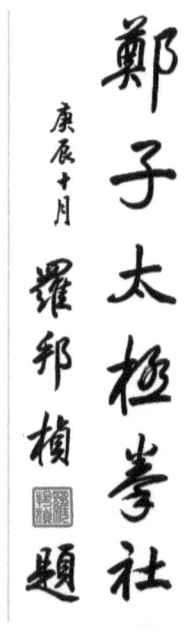

What is Tai Chi Chuan?

Tai Chi Chuan is an internal Chinese martial art, often promoted and practiced as a martial arts therapy for the purposes of health and longevity. Tai Chi Chuan is considered a soft style martial art, an art applied with as much deep relaxation or softness in the musculature as possible, to distinguish its theory and application from that of the hard martial art styles which use a degree of tension in the muscles.

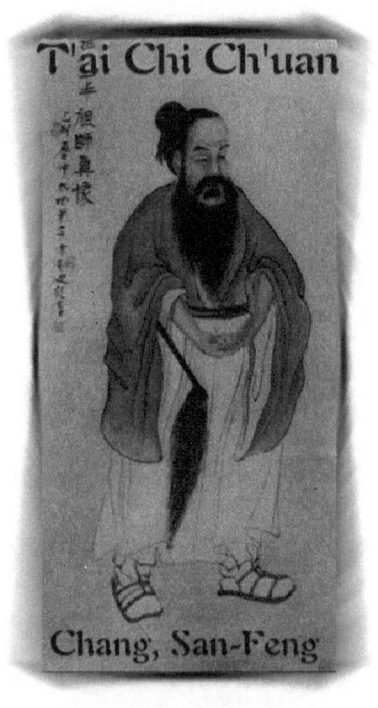

T'ai Chi Ch'uan

Chang, San-Feng

Variations of basic training forms are well known as the slow motion routines that groups of people practice every morning in parks across China and other parts of the world.

Traditional Tai Chi training is intended to teach awareness of one's own balance and what affects it, awareness of the same in others, an appreciation of the practical value in one's ability to moderate extremes of behavior and attitude at both mental and physical levels, and how this applies to effective self-defense principles.

Based on softness and awareness, rather than force and resistance, Tai Chi Chuan has been recognized for thousands of years as both a method of self-cultivation and an unexcelled form of self-defense.

The Movements

Tai Chi Chuan is a noncompetitive, self-paced system of gentle physical exercise and stretching. You perform a series of postures or movements in a slow, graceful manner. Each posture flows into the next without pausing. Anyone, regardless of age or physical ability, can practice these movements as they require awareness rather than strength, and they can be done effortlessly. It doesn't take physical prowess.

The Benefits

- Reduce stress

- Increase flexibility

- Improve muscle strength and definition

- Increase energy, stamina and agility

- Increase your general sense of wellbeing

Tai Chi Chuan knows more than one hundred possible movements and positions. You can find several that you like, and stick with those, or explore the full range. The intensity of the movements varies somewhat depending on the form or style practiced. Some forms are more fast-paced than others, for instance. However, most forms are gentle and suitable for everyone. And they all include *rhythmic patterns of movement* that are to be coordinated with breathing.

Like other practices that bring mind and body together, the practice of Tai Chi Chuan reduces stress. When you do the movements, you focus on movement and breathing. This combination creates a state of relaxation and calm. Stress, anxiety and tension should melt away as you focus on the present, and the effects may last well after you stop your session.

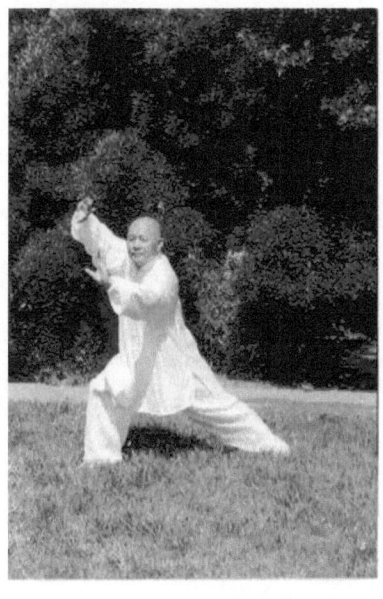

Tai Chi Chuan may also help your overall health, although it's not a substitute for traditional medical care, but rather a form of prophylaxis. Tai Chi Chuan is generally safe for people of all ages and levels of fitness. Older adults may especially find it appealing because the movements are low impact and put minimal stress on muscles and joints. Tai Chi Chuan may also be helpful if you have arthritis or are recovering from an injury.

Learning the Technique

Wondering how to get started? You don't need any special clothing or equipment. To gain full benefits, however, it may be best to seek guidance from a qualified instructor, who can teach you specific positions and how to regulate your breathing. An instructor also can teach you how to practice safely, especially if you have injuries, chronic conditions, or balance or coordination problems.

Practice Regularly

To reap the greatest stress reduction benefits from Tai Chi Chuan, consider practicing it regularly. Many people find it helpful to practice in the same place and at the same time every day to develop a routine. But if your schedule is erratic, do your cycle whenever you have a few minutes. You can even draw on the soothing concepts of Tai Chi Chuan without performing the actual movements if you get stuck in stressful situations — a traffic jam or a work conflict, for instance. You can do your movements in your mind, for example, remembering the feelings of wellbeing that you experienced when doing it last time. The Tai Chi Chuan movements are widely acknowledged to help calm the emotions, focus the mind, and strengthen the immune system. In a very real sense, it helps us to stay younger as we grow older, thus making an outstanding contribution to our overall health and wellbeing.

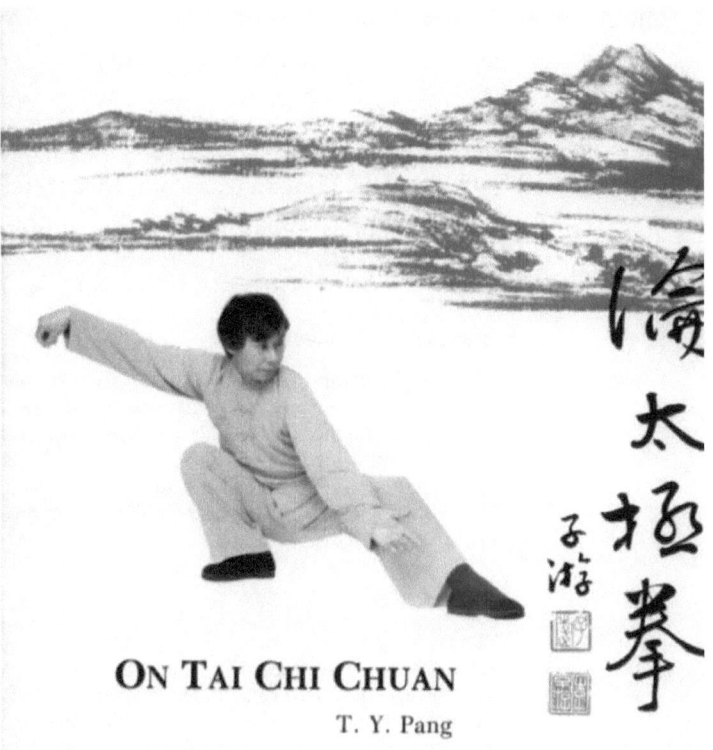

ON TAI CHI CHUAN

T. Y. Pang

Meaning of the Word

The term *Tai Chi Chuan* literally translates as 'supreme ultimate fist', 'boundless fist', 'great extremes boxing', or simply 'the ultimate'. Tai Chi Chuan is generally classified as a form of traditional Chinese martial arts of the soft or internal branch. It is considered a soft style martial art, an art applied with internal power, to distinguish its theory and application from that of the hard martial art styles.

Tai Chi Chuan, by Master Shou-Yu Liang

This is a review of Master Liang's outstanding book and DVD entitled *Tai Chi Chuan, 24 & 48 Postures with Martial Applications*, Roslindale: YMAA Publication Center, 1996. Before I purchased book and DVD on amazon.com, I was reading to of the reviews, and publish them here, as I find them well-written and to the point:

Midwest Book Review

One of China's top-ranked coaches to Tai Chi provides an illustrated guide to the 24 and 48 postures, including tips on breathing, aligning the body, and developing Chi. Martial applications are also surveyed in a presentation notable for its many step-by-step black and white photos which excel in illustrating positions and movements.

Duane

The simplified, widely practiced 24-posture form was devised by the Chinese government in the 1950's due to a shortage of doctors. Founded primarily on the Yang style, it takes 5-10 minutes to practice, less time than for the 37- and 108-posture forms.

Yang style is probably the most thoroughly documented style of Taijiquan, for better or worse. So this 24-posture short version represents a mainstream starting point.

Liang's compact manual probably offers the most complete and concise description of this form available, together with overview of historical background, training tips, and illustrations of martial applications "hidden" within the form.

The companion video of the same name (purchased separately) shows the sequence twice from the front view, once from the back. Then it shows martial applications individually and also the 48-posture version.

To get the 24-posture form broken down in detail, I also recommend Dr. Paul Lam's DVD, 'Tai Chi the 24 forms'.

In the YMAA tradition of Dr. Yang, this manual (and video) represent training notes at a disciplined, somewhat demanding level. The numbering system for the photographs, together with the compactness of the page layout have caused me to pencil in some arrows and titles.

If you're simply looking for a group stretching routine to follow along with at your local community center, you may consider this text ambitious.

It was the above-quoted book review by Mr. C. Duane, that is published on amazon.com that gave the trigger to my buying this book, and the corresponding DVD.

I was positively surprised when I received the book and DVD. What I found especially useful are the black arrows that trace all the movements to be made. In addition, you see them performed by Master Liang on the DVD, and further, there is a meticulous description simultaneous to the movements, in English, to be heard on the DVD. I can't imagine how to do it better; this is simply the best form of pedagogy for learning Tai Chi – which is if you want to do it in the right way, not in the Western way, *not easy* to learn. It requires full attention to detail and a fully developed body consciousness. And that is exactly what it develops in the first place. It raises our body consciousness or what I came to term *emonic consciousness*, because it implies awareness of the *ch'i*, the vital energy flow in the organism. The author introduces the book with the following elucidation that I think is worth to be quoted:

Master Liang

Chinese view the universe as one interrelated organism, not as separate entities; everything resonates with each other to reach balance and harmony. This view, on a smaller scale, also applies to the human body. It is believed that studying the universe will give us an understanding of the small universe - the human body./2

Indeed, what our new science is now discovering, and I refer you here only to the books of Ervin Laszlo and Rupert Sheldrake that I reviewed in my *110 Book Reviews (2010)*, was known to the Chinese already more than five thousand years ago. So there is nothing new under the sun, in fact. The only difference between ancient China and our times in this context is the fact that they called knowledge philosophy, while we call it science, but these expressions actually mean the same.

And the parallel goes even farther. The ancient Chinese sages knew that knowledge alone, as long as it's mere theory or concepts, will not really foster human evolution; what is further needed is to align our breath with the cosmic breath, and this was done, in China, through Qigong, and Tai Chi Chuan. All Eastern martial arts are in essence breathing exercises; all movements are done with the ultimate purpose of teaching us how to breathe properly. And in the West, many managers and high-grade officials have discovered in a process that goes over the last two or three decades that knowledge and skills alone will not make a really powerful, effective, human, and wistful manager. And that is why, naturally, managers and leaders from all walks of life nowadays discover *mindbody coordinating techniques,* such as Zen, Qigong and Tai Chi Chuan, and some others.

There is a fast growing awareness since the 1990s that these techniques actually are a must for whoever is in a position of leading others, for moral integrity is one of the finest elements of these techniques since the oldest traditions, as it was known since the beginnings of human history that a good leader can only be one who has achieved moral integrity at a high and even outstanding level.

What is this moral integrity about? Beware, it is not what I came to call *moralism*, and it is not judging others and life, it is not persecuting others because they have different sexual tastes, and it is not splitting life in a good-and-bad scheme. It is *true* morality, not the fake many Westerners are addicted to and that they call 'good behavior' or 'decency'. It is nothing of all that. It is integrity, and acceptance; it is intelligent and non-judgmental understanding at a very high level. It is also compassion, empathy with self and others, tolerance, and emotional maturity.

Master Liang says that training the mind is of the highest importance for the practice of Tai Chi Chuan. And this is naturally so because what happens when we train the mind is that we *build awareness of our projections* that grow out from our blind spots and moral weaknesses. Master Liang formulates moral integrity in these rather pragmatic terms:

Master Liang

To achieve the maximum benefit from Taijiquan practice, you should 'practice Taijiquan 24 hours a day'. This doesn't mean that you need to do the Taijiquan sequence all the time, but you need to make Taijiquan a way of life. The practice of Taijiquan will not only provide a 'whole' body workout; but also cultivate the energy within your body, increase your mental awareness and centering, and build good habits for proper body alignment. When you have accomplished these goals in practice, you will automatically carry these good habits into your daily life. You will gain a greater awareness of yourself; keeping your physical body properly aligned while sitting, standing, driving, eating, watching TV, working, typing, brushing your teeth, and everything else you do regularly. This is what is meant by 'practicing Taijiquan 24 hours a day' and 'making Taijiquan a way of life'./15

Now to come to the practical part of the book, let me say that I found it a bit 'upside down' that the book commences with the preparatory Qigong techniques and then jumps to difficult martial art stances for accomplished masters; only after that comes in Chapter Five and on page 95 to the daily 48 Postures Tai Chi Chuan that most of us practice. If that was voluntary on the part of the authors, and it certainly was, the reason for this escapes me. And by the way, on the DVD, it's in the same order.

TIBETAN MEDICINE

Feeling the Pulse

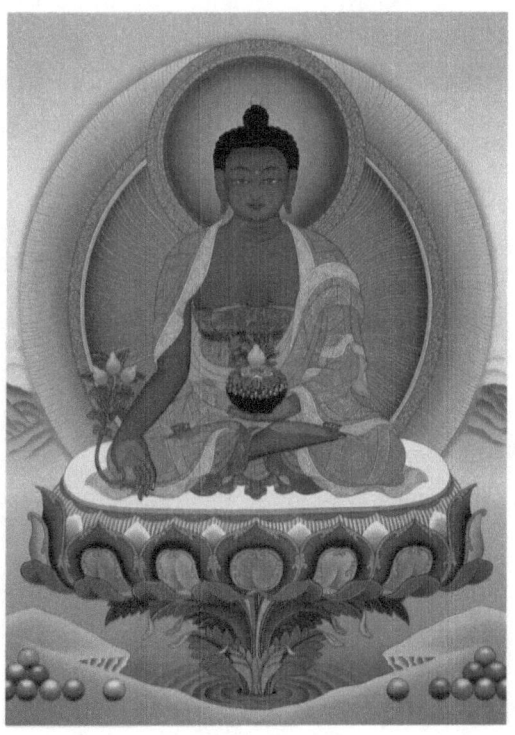

I discovered Tibetan traditional medicine in 1994, in the Netherlands. I had suffered from a long-lasting pain in my right knee that no Western doctor could heal, and my Chinese friends in Rotterdam sent me to a Tibetan healer in Amsterdam.

While all the Western doctors had diagnosed some or the other local problem with the ligaments, the Tibetan healer, after feeling my pulse for quite a long moment, said there was nothing wrong with my knee's ligaments, and the problem was instead a *cold spot* that probably was caused through uncovering myself during sleep.

I was rather suspicious to this diagnosis as it sounded so simplistic, but followed the advice of the healer to wear a *simple woolen bandage* around the knee for a minimum of two weeks.

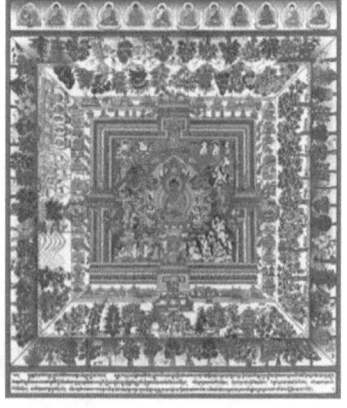

In addition, he gave me a herbal balm that was, as he said, keeping my knee warm, and advised me to once in a while take a warm bath. To my surprise, after two or three weeks, the pain was gone and was never any more coming up thereafter.

And the doctor, despite my insisting upon paying his fee, refused to accept any payment, despite the fact that in addition to one hour of consultation, he had given me the balm and the woolen bandage for free.

As I had been recommended by friends, he explained, he was not supposed to accept any payment. I did not need further elucidation about the *professional ethics,* the competence and the supreme level of virtue of Tibetan natural healers.

YOGA

The Two Yoga

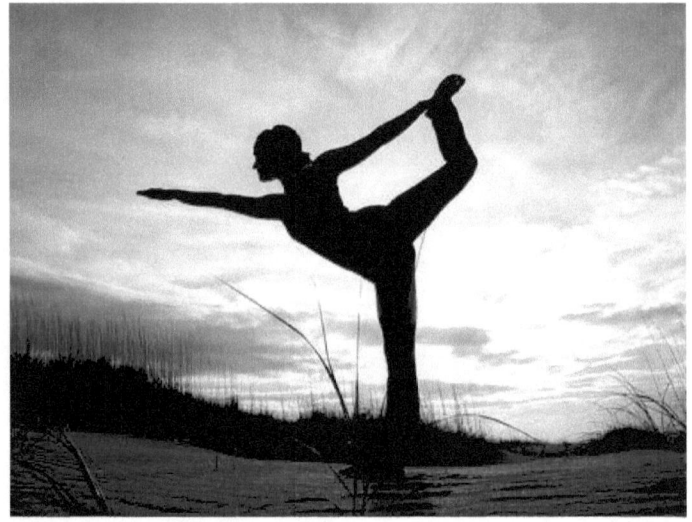

Indian Yoga

The word Yoga means to join or unite. It is generally translated as union of the individual *atman* or individual soul with *paramatman* or *brahman* or universal soul.

Yoga is a family of ancient spiritual practices dating back more than five thousand years from India. It is one of the six schools of Hindu philosophy.

In India, Yoga is seen as a means to both physiological and spiritual mastery. Outside of India, Yoga has become primarily associated with the practice of *asanas (postures)* of Hatha Yoga.

Yoga as a means of spiritual attainment is central to Hinduism, Buddhism and Jainism and has influenced other religious and spiritual practices throughout the world. Hindu texts establishing the basis for yoga include the *Upanishads*, the *Bhagavad Gita*, the *Yoga Sutras of Patanjali*, the *Hatha Yoga Pradipika* and many others. The four main paths of Yoga are *Karma Yoga, Jnana Yoga, Bhakti Yoga* and *Raja Yoga*. Practitioners of yoga are referred to as a *yogi* or *yogin* (male), and *yogini* (female).

Chinese-Thai Yoga

Tao Yoga is a method coined by the Thai-American Master Mantak Chia that consists in directing the bioenergetic flow of the organism by means of mental focus and deep breathing. Mantak Chia has explained and illustrated the method and its application extensively in his books.

BIBLIOGRAPHY

General Bibliography

A

Abrams, Jeremiah (Ed.)
Reclaiming the Inner Child
New York: Tarcher/Putnam, 1990

Die Befreiung des Inneren Kindes
Die Wiederentdeckung unserer ursprünglichen kreativen Persönlichkeit
und ihre zentrale Bedeutung für unser Erwachsenwerden
München: Scherz Verlag, 1993

Adrienne, Carol
The Numerology Kit
New American Library, 1988

Agni Yoga Society
COEUR : Signes de l'Agni Yoga
Toulon: Sté Edipub, 1985
Publication originale date de 1932

Albrecht, Karl
The Only Thing That Matters
New York: Harper & Row, 1993

Alston, John P. / Tucker, Francis
The Myth of Sexual Permissiveness
The Journal of Sex Research, 9/1 (1973)

Appleton, Matthew
A Free Range Childhood
Self-Regulation at Summerhill School
Foundation for Educational Renewal, 2000

Summerhill
Kindern ihre Kindheit zurückgeben
Demokratie und Selbstregulierung in der Erziehung
Hohengehren: Schneider Verlag, 2003

Arcas, Gérald, Dr

Guérir le corps par l'hypnose et l'auto-hypnose
Paris: Sand, 1997

Ariès, Philippe

L'enfant et la famille sous l'Ancien Régime
Paris, Seuil, 1975

Centuries of Childhood
New York: Vintage Books, 1962

Geschichte der Kindheit
Frankfurt/M: DTV, 1998

Arntz, William & Chasse, Betsy

What the Bleep Do We Know
20th Century Fox, 2005 (DVD)

Down The Rabbit Hole Quantum Edition
20th Century Fox, 2006 (3 DVD Set)

Bleep
An der Schnittstelle von Spiritualität und Wissenschaft
Verblüffende Erkenntnisse und Anstösse zum Weiterdenken
Berlin: Vak Verlag, 2007

Arroyo, Stephen

Astrology, Karma & Transformation
The Inner Dimensions of the Birth Chart
Sebastopol, CA: CRSC Publications, 1978

Astrologie, Karma und Transformation
Die Chancen schwieriger Aspekte
Frankfurt/M: Heyne Verlag, 1998

Relationships and Life Cycles
Astrological Patterns of Personal Experience
Sebastopol, CA: CRCS Publications, 1993

Handbuch der Horoskop-Deutung
Berlin: Rowohlt, 1999

B

Bachelard, Gaston

The Poetics of Reverie
Translated by Daniel Russell
Boston: Beacon Press, 1971

Poetik des Raumes
Frankfurt/M: Fischer Verlag, 2001

Bandler, Richard

Get the Life You Want
The Secrets to Quick and Lasting Life Change
With Neuro-Linguistic Programming
Deerfield Beach, Fl: HCI, 2008

Barron, Frank X., Montuori, et al. (Eds.)

Creators on Creating
Awakening and Cultivating the Imaginative Mind
(New Consciousness Reader)
New York: P. Tarcher/Putnam, 1997

Bertalanffy, Ludwig von

General Systems Theory
Foundations, Development, Applications
New York: George Brazilier Publishing, 1976

Besant, Annie

An Autobiography
New Delhi: Penguin Books, 2005
Originally published in 1893

Karma
4e édition
Paris: Adyar, 1923

Bettelheim, Bruno

A Good Enough Parent
New York: A. Knopf, 1987

The Uses of Enchantment
New York: Vintage Books, 1989

Kinder brauchen Märchen
Frankfurt/M: DTV, 2002

Block, Peter

Stewardship
Choosing Service Over Self-Interest
San Francisco: Berrett-Koehler, 1996

Blofeld, J.

The Book of Changes
A New Translation of the Ancient Chinese I Ching
New York: E.P. Dutton, 1965

Blum, Ralph H. & Laughan, Susan

The Healing Runes
Tools for the Recovery of Body, Mind, Heart & Soul
New York: St. Martin's Press, 1995

Boadalla, David

Wilhelm Reich, Leben und Werk
Frankfurt/M: Fischer, 1980

Böhm, Wilfried

Maria Montessori
2. Auflage
Bad Heilbrunn: Julius Klinkhardt, 1991

Bohm, David

Wholeness and the Implicate Order
London: Routledge, 2002

Die implizite Ordnung
Grundlagen eines dynamischen Holismus
München: Goldmann Wilhelm, 1989

Thought as a System
London: Routledge, 1994

Quantum Theory
London: Dover Publications, 1989

La plénitude de l'univers
Paris: Rocher, 1992

La conscience de l'univers
Paris: Rocher, 1992

Boldt, Laurence G.

Zen and the Art of Making a Living
A Practical Guide to Creative Career Design
New York: Penguin Arkana, 1993

How to Find the Work You Love
New York: Penguin Arkana, 1996

Zen Soup
Tasty Morsels of Zen Wisdom From Great Minds East & West
New York: Penguin Arkana, 1997

The Tao of Abundance
Eight Ancient Principles For Abundant Living

New York: Penguin Arkana, 1999

Das Tao der Fülle
Vom Reichtum, der uns glücklich macht
Mittelberg: Joy Verlag, 2001

Bordeaux-Szekely, Edmond

*Teaching of the Essenes from Enoch to the Dead
Sea Scrolls*
Beekman Publishing, 1992

Gospel of the Essenes
The Unknown Books of the Essenes
& Lost Scrolls of the Essene Brotherhood
Beekman Publishing, 1988

Gospel of Peace of Jesus Christ
Beekman Publishing, 1994

Gospel of Peace, 2d Vol.
I B S International Publishers

Das Friedensevangelium der Essener
Saarbrücken: Neue Erde/Lentz, 2002

Évangile essénien de la paix
La vie biogénique
Genève: Éditions Soleil, 1978

Die unbekannten Schriften der Essener
Saarbrücken: Neue Erde/Lentz, 2002

Branden, Nathaniel

How to Raise Your Self-Esteem
New York: Bantam, 1987

Die 6 Säulen des Selbstwertgefühls
Erfolgreich und zufrieden durch ein starkes Selbst
München: Piper Verlag, 2009

Brennan, Barbara Ann

Hands of Healing
A Guide to Healing Through the Human Energy Field
New York: Bantam, 1988

Bullough & Bullough (Eds.)

Human Sexuality
An Encyclopedia
New York: Garland Publishing, 1994

Sin, Sickness and Sanity
A History of Sexual Attitudes
New York: New American Library, 1977

Butler-Bowden, Tom

50 Success Classics
Winning Wisdom for Work & Life From 50 Landmark Books
London: Nicholas Brealey Publishing, 2004

50 Klassiker des Erfolgs
Die wichtigsten Werke von Kenneth Blanchard, Warren Buffet,
Andrew Carnegie, Stephen R. Covey, Spencer Johnson,
Benjamin Franklin, Napoleon Hill, Nelson Mandela, Anthony Robbins,
Brian Tracy, Sun Tsu, Jack Welch und vielen anderen
Frankfurt/M: MVG Verlag, 2005

50 Lebenshilfe Klassiker
Frankfurt/M: MVG Verlag, 2004

50 Klassiker der Psychologie
Die wichtigsten Werke von Alfred Adler, Sigmund Freud,
Daniel Goleman, Karen Horney, William James, C.G. Jung, Jean Piaget,
Viktor Frankl, Howard Gardner, Alfred Kinsey, Abraham Maslow, Iwan
Pawlow, Stanley Milgram, Martin Seligman und vielen anderen
Frankfurt/M: MVG Verlag, 2004

50 Klassiker der Spiritualität
Die wichtigsten Werke von Augustinus, Khalil Gibran, Mahatma Ghandi,
Dag Hammarskjölkd, Hermann Hesse, C. G. Jung, Eckhart Tolle,

J. Krishnamurti, Thich Nhat Hanh, Mutter Teresa, Dan Millman
und vielen anderen
Frankfurt/M: MVG Verlag, 2006

C

Cain, Chelsea & Moon Unit Zappa

Wild Child
New York: Seal Press (Feminist Publishing), 1999

Calderone & Ramey

Talking With Your Child About Sex
New York: Random House, 1982

Campbell, Herbert James

The Pleasure Areas
London: Eyre Methuen Ltd., 1973

Der Irrtum mit der Seele
München: Scherz Verlag, 1973

Les principes du plaisir
Paris: Stock, 1974

Capacchione, Lucia

The Power of Your Other Hand
North Hollywood, CA: Newcastle Publishing, 1988

Capra, Fritjof

The Turning Point
Science, Society And The Rising Culture
New York: Simon & Schuster, 1987
Original Author Copyright, 1982

Wendezeit
Bausteine für ein neues Weltbild
München: Droemer Knaur, 2004

Le temps du changement
Science, société et nouvelle culture
Paris: Rocher, 1994

The Tao of Physics
An Exploration of the Parallels Between Modern
Physics and Eastern Mysticism
New York: Shambhala Publications, 2000
(New Edition) Originally published in 1975

Das Tao der Physik
Die Konvergenz von westlicher Wissenschaft und östlicher Philosophie
Neue und erweiterte Auflage
München: O.W. Barth bei Scherz, 2000
Ursprünglich erschienen 1975 bei Droemersche Verlagsanstalt
in Hamburg

Le tao de la physique
Paris: Sand & Tchou, 1994

The Web of Life
A New Scientific Understanding of Living Systems
New York: Doubleday, 1997
Author Copyright 1996

Lebensnetz
Ein neues Verständnis der lebendigen Welt
München: Scherz Verlag, 1999

The Hidden Connections
Integrating The Biological, Cognitive And Social
Dimensions Of Life Into A Science Of Sustainability
New York: Doubleday, 2002

Verborgene Zusammenhänge
München: Scherz, 2002

Steering Business Toward Sustainability
New York: United Nations University Press, 1995

Uncommon Wisdom
Conversations with Remarkable People
New York: Bantam, 1989

The Science of Leonardo
Inside the Mind of the Great Genius of the Renaissance
New York: Anchor Books, 2008
New York: Bantam Doubleday, 2007 (First Publishing)

Complete List of Publications
http://www.fritjofcapra.net/publishers.html

Cassou, Michelle & Cubley, Steward

Life, Paint and Passion
Reclaiming the Magic of Spontaneous Expression
New York: P. Tarcher/Putnam, 1996

Castaneda, Carlos

The Teachings of Don Juan
A Yaqui Way of Knowledge
Washington: Square Press, 1985

Journey to Ixtlan
Washington: Square Press: 1991

Tales of Power
Washington: Square Press, 1991

The Second Ring of Power
Washington: Square Press, 1991

Castel, Robert

L'ordre psychiatrique, l'âge d'or de l'aliénisme
Paris: Éditions de Minuit, 1977

Chopra, Deepak

Creating Affluence
The A-to-Z Steps to a Richer Life
New York: Amber-Allen Publishing (2003)

Life After Death
The Book of Answers
London: Rider, 2006

Leben nach dem Tod
Das letzte Geheimnis unserer Existenz
Berlin: Allegria Verlag, 2008

Synchrodestiny
Discover the Power of Meaningful Coincidence to Manifest Abundance
Audio Book / CD
Niles, IL: Nightingale-Conant, 2006

The Seven Spiritual Laws of Success
A Practical Guide to the Fulfillment of Your Dreams
Audio Book / CD
New York: Amber-Allen Publishing (2002)

Die Sieben Geistigen Gesetze des Erfolgs
Berlin: Ullstein Verlag, 2004

The Spontaneous Fulfillment of Desire
Harnessing the Infinite Power of Coincidence
New York: Random House Audio, 2003

Cleary, Thomas

The Taoist I Ching
Translated by Thomas Cleary
Boston & London: Shambhala, 1986

Covey, Stephen R.

The 7 Habits of Highly Effective People
Powerful Lessons in Personal Change
New York: Free Press, 2004

15th Anniversary Edition
First Published in 1989

Die 7 Wege zur Effektivität
Prinzipien für persönlichen und beruflichen Erfolg
Offenbach: Gabal Verlag, 2009

The 8th Habit
From Effectiveness to Greatness
London: Simon & Schuster, 2004

Der 8. Weg
Von der Effektivität zur wahren Grösse
Offenbach: Gabal Verlag, 2006

D

De Bono, Edward

The Use of Lateral Thinking
New York: Penguin, 1967

The Mechanism of Mind
New York: Penguin, 1969

Sur/Petition
London: HarperCollins, 1993

Tactics
London: HarperCollins, 1993
First published in 1985

Taktiken und Strategien erfolgreicher Menschen
Frankfurt/M: MVG Verlag, 1995

Serious Creativity
Using the Power of Lateral Thinking to Create New Ideas
London: HarperCollins, 1996

Deshimaru, Taisen

Zen et vie quotidienne
Paris: Albin Michel, 1985

Diamond, Stephen A., May, Rollo

Anger, Madness, and the Daimonic
The Psychological Genesis of Violence, Evil and Creativity
New York: State University of New York Press, 1999

DiCarlo, Russell E. (Ed.)

Towards A New World View
Conversations at the Leading Edge
Erie, PA: Epic Publishing, 1996

Dürckheim, Karlfried Graf

Hara: The Vital Center of Man
Rochester: Inner Traditions, 2004

Hara
Die Erdmitte des Menschen
Neuausgabe
München: O.W. Barth bei Scherz, 2005

Zen and Us
New York: Penguin Arkana 1991

The Call for the Master
New York: Penguin Books, 1993

Absolute Living
The Otherworldly in the World and the Path to Maturity
New York: Penguin Arkana, 1992

The Way of Transformation
Daily Life as a Spiritual Exercise
London: Allen & Unwin, 1988

Der Alltag als Übung
Vom Weg der Verwandlung
Bern: Huber, 2008

The Japanese Cult of Tranquility
London: Rider, 1960

Kultur der Stille
Frankfurt/M: Weltz Verlag, 1997

E

Eden, Donna & Feinstein, David

Energy Medicine
New York: Tarcher/Putnam, 1998

The Energy Medicine Kit
Simple Effective Techniques to Help You Boost Your Vitality
Boulder, Co.: Sounds True Editions, 2004

The Promise of Energy Psychology
With David Feinstein and Gary Craig
Revolutionary Tools for Dramatic Personal Change
New York: Jeremy P. Tarcher/Penguin, 2005

Edmunds, Francis

An Introduction to Anthroposophy
Rudolf Steiner's Worldview
London: Rudolf Steiner Press, 2005

Emoto, Masaru

The Hidden Messages in Water
New York: Atria Books, 2004

Die Botschaft des Wassers
Burgrain: Koha Verlag, 2008

The Secret Life of Water
New York: Atria Books, 2005

Die Heilkraft des Wassers
Burgrain: Koha Verlag, 2004

Erickson, Milton H.

My Voice Will Go With You
The Teaching Tales of Milton H. Erickson
by Sidney Rosen (Ed.)
New York: Norton & Co., 1991

Complete Works 1.0, CD-ROM
New York: Milton H. Erickson Foundation, 2001

Erikson, Erik H.

Childhood and Society
New York: Norton, 1993
First published in 1950

F

Fensterhalm, Herbert

Don't Say Yes When You Want to Say No
With Jean Bear
New York: Dell, 1980

Flack, Audrey

Art & Soul
Notes on Creating
New York: E P Dutton, Reissue Edition, 1991

Foucault, Michel

The History of Sexuality, Vol. I : The Will to Knowledge
London: Penguin, 1998
First published in 1976

The History of Sexuality, Vol. II : The Use of Pleasure
London: Penguin, 1998
First published in 1984

The History of Sexuality, Vol. III : The Care of Self
London: Penguin, 1998
First published in 1984

Fourcade, Jean-Michel

Analyse transactionnelle et bioénergie
Paris: Delarge, 1981

Franz Anton Mesmer

Franz Anton Mesmer und die Geschichte des Mesmerismus
Beiträge zum internationalen wissenschaftlichen Symposium
anlässlich des 250. Geburtstages von Mesmer
Stuttgart, 1985

Freud, Sigmund

Three Essays on the Theory of Sexuality
in: The Standard Edition of the Complete Psychological
Works of Sigmund Freud
London: Hogarth Press, 1953-54
Vol. 7, pp. 130 ff
(first published in 1905)

Drei Abhandlungen zur Sexualtheorie
Frankfurt/M: Fischer, 1991

The Interpretation of Dreams
New York: Avon, Reissue Edition, 1980
and in: The Standard Edition of the Complete Psychological
Works of Sigmund Freud , (24 Volumes) ed. by James Strachey
New York: W. W. Norton & Company, 1976

Die Traumdeutung
Frankfurt/M: Fischer, 2005

Totem and Taboo
New York: Routledge, 1999
Originally published in 1913

Totem und Tabu
Einige Übereinstimmungen im Seelenleben der Wilden und
der Neurotiker
Frankfurt/M: Fischer Verlag, 1972

Fromm, Erich

The Anatomy of Human Destructiveness
New York: Owl Book, 1992
Originally published in 1973

Anatomie der menschlichen Destruktivität
Berlin: Rowohlt, 1977

Escape from Freedom
New York: Owl Books, 1994
Originally published in 1941

Die Furcht vor der Freiheit
München: DTV Verlag, 1993

To Have or To Be
New York: Continuum International Publishing, 1996
Originally published in 1976

Haben oder Sein
Die seelischen Grundlagen einer neuen Gesellschaft
München: DTV Verlag, 2005

The Art of Loving
New York: HarperPerennial, 2000
Originally published in 1956

Die Kunst des Liebens
Berlin: Ullstein, 2005

G

Gawain, Shakti

Creative Visualization
Use the Power of Your Imagination to Create What You Want
Novato, CA: New World Library, 1995

Creative Visualization Meditations (Reader)
Novato, CA: New World Library, 1997

Geldard, Richard

Remembering Heraclitus
New York: Lindisfarne Books, 2000

Gerber, Richard

A Practical Guide to Vibrational Medicine
Energy Healing and Spiritual Transformation
New York: Harper & Collins, 2001

Geller, Uri

The Mindpower Kit
Includes Book, Audiotape, Quartz Crystal And Meditation Circle
New York: Penguin, 1996

Gesell, Izzy

Playing Along
37 Group Learning Activities Borrowed from Improvisational Theater
Whole Person Associates, 1997

Ghiselin, Brewster (Ed.)

The Creative Process
Reflections on Invention in the Arts and Sciences
Berkeley: University of California Press, 1985
First published in 1952

Goldman, Jonathan & Goldman, Andi

Tantra of Sound
Frequencies of Healing
Charlottesville: Hampton Roads, 2005

Tantra des Klanges
Mehr Liebe und Intimität in der Partnerschaft
Mit CD
Hanau: Amra Verlag, 2009

Healing Sounds
The Power of Harmonies
Rochester: Healing Arts Press, 2002

Klangheilung
Die Schöpferkraft des Obertongesangs
Hanau: Amra Verlag, 2008

Healing Sounds
Principles of Sound Healing
DVD, 90 min.
Sacred Mysteries, 2004

Goleman, Daniel

Emotional Intelligence
New York, Bantam Books, 1995

EQ. Emotionale Intelligenz
München: DTV Verlag, 1997

Goswami, Amit

The Self-Aware Universe
How Consciousness Creates the Material World
New York: Tarcher/Putnam, 1995

Das Bewusste Universum
Wie Bewusstsein die materielle Welt erschafft
Stuttgart: Lüchow Verlag, 2007

Grant

Grant's Method of Anatomy
10th ed., by John V. Basmajian
Baltimore, London: Williams & Wilkins, 1980

Greene, Liz

Astrology of Fate
York Beach, ME: Red Wheel/Weiser, 1986

Saturn
A New Look at an Old Devil
York Beach, ME: Red Wheel/Weiser, 1976

The Astrological Neptune and the Quest for Redemption
Boston: Red Wheel Weiser, 1996

The Mythic Journey
With Juliet Sharman-Burke
The Meaning of Myth as a Guide for Life
New York: Simon & Schuster (Fireside), 2000

Die Mythische Reise
Die Bedeutung der Mythen als ein Führer durch das Leben
München: Atmosphären Verlag, 2004

The Mythic Tarot
With Juliet Sharman-Burke
New York: Simon & Schuster (Fireside), 2001
Originally published in 1986

Le Tarot Mythique
Une nouvelle approche du Tarot
Paris: Solar, 1988

The Luminaries
The Psychology of the Sun and Moon in the Horoscope
With Howard Sasportas
York Beach, ME: Red Wheel/Weiser, 1992

Sonne und Mond
Die Bedeutung der grossen Lichter in der Mythologie und im Horoskop
Saarbrücken: Neue Erde/Lentz, 2000

Grinspoon, Lester

Marihuana
The Forbidden Medicine
With James B. Bakalar
New Haven, CT: Yale University Press, 1997
First published in 1971

Grof, Stanislav

Ancient Wisdom and Modern Science
New York: State University of New York Press, 1984

Beyond the Brain
Birth, Death and Transcendence in Psychotherapy
New York: State University of New York, 1985

LSD: Doorway to the Numinous
The Groundbreaking Psychedelic Research into Realms of the
Human Unconscious
Rochester: Park Street Press, 2009

Psychologie transpersonnelle
Paris: Rocher, 1984

Realms of the Human Unconscious
Observations from LSD Research
New York: E.P. Dutton, 1976

The Cosmic Game
Explorations of the Frontiers of Human Consciousness
New York: State University of New York Press, 1998

The Holotropic Mind
The Three Levels of Human Consciousness
With Hal Zina Bennett
New York: HarperCollins, 1993

When the Impossible Happens
Adventures in Non-Ordinary Reality
Louisville, CO: Sounds True, 2005

Wir wissen mehr als unser Gehirn
Die Grenzen des Bewusstseins überschreiten
Freiburg: Herder, 2007

Groth, A. Nicholas

Men Who Rape
The Psychology of the Offender
New York: Perseus Publishing, 1980

Grout, Pam

Art & Soul
New York: Andrews McMeel Publishing, 2000

Gurdjieff, George Ivanovich

The Herald of Coming Good
London: Samuel Weiser, 1933

H

Hall, Manly P.

The Pineal Gland
The Eye of God
Article extracted from the book: Man the Grand Symbol of the Mysteries
Kessinger Publishing Reprint

The Secret Teachings of All Ages
Reader's Edition
New York: Tarcher/Penguin, 2003
Originally published in 1928

Harner, Michael

Ways of the Shaman
New York: Bantam, 1982
Originally published in 1980

Der Weg des Schamanen
Das praktische Grundlagenbuch zum Schamanismus
Genf: Ariston, 2007

Chamane
Les secrets d'un sorcier indien d'Amérique du Nord
Paris: Albin Michel, 1982

Hermes Trismegistos

Corpus Hermeticum
New York: Edaf, 2001

Herrigel, Eugen

Zen in the Art of Archery
New York: Vintage Books, 1999
Originally published in 1971

Hicks, Esther and Jerry

The Amazing Power of Deliberate Intent
Living the Art of Allowing
Carlsbad, CA: Hay House, 2006

Hofmann, Albert

LSD, My Problem Child
Reflections on Sacred Drugs, Mysticism and Science
Santa Cruz, CA: Multidisciplinary Association for Psychedelic Studies, 2009
Originally published in 1980

LSD, Mein Sorgenkind
Die Entdeckung der 'Wunderdroge'
München: DTV Verlag, 1999

Holmes, Ernst

The Science of Mind
A Philosophy, A Faith, A Way of Life
New York: Jeremy P. Tarcher/Putnam, 1998
First Published in 1938

Holstiege, Hildegard

Montessori Pädagogik und soziale Humanität
Freiburg: Herder, 1994

Hood, J. X.

Scientific Curiosities of Love, Sex and Marriage
A Survey of Sex Relations, Beliefs and Customs of Mankind in
Different Countries and Ages
New York, 1951

Houston, Jean

The Possible Human
A Course in Enhancing Your Physical, Mental, and Creative Abilities
New York: Jeremy P. Tarcher/Putnam, 1982

Huang, Alfred

The Complete I Ching
The Definite Translation from Taoist Master Alfred Huang
Rochester, NY: Inner Traditions, 1998

Hunt, Valerie

Infinite Mind
Science of the Human Vibrations of Consciousness
Malibu, CA: Malibu Publishing, 2000

Huxley, Aldous

The Doors of Perception and Heaven and Hell
London: HarperCollins (Flamingo), 1994
(originally published in 1954)

The Perennial Philosophy
San Francisco: Harper & Row, 1970

J

James, William

Writings 1902-1910
The Varieties of Religious Experience / Pragmatism / A Pluralistic
Universe / The Meaning of Truth / Some Problems of Philosophy / Essays
New York: Library of America, 1988

Jampolsky, Gerald

Aimer c'est se libérer de la peur
Genève: Éditions Soleil, 1986

Janov, Arthur

Primal Man
The New Consciousness
New York: Crowell, 1975

Das Neue Bewusstsein
Frankfurt/M: Fischer Verlag, 1988
Urausgabe 1975

Jung, Carl Gustav

Archetypen
München: DTV Verlag, 2001

Archetypes of the Collective Unconscious
in: The Basic Writings of C.G. Jung
New York: The Modern Library, 1959, 358-407

Collected Works
New York, 1959

Dialectique du moi et de l'inconscient
Paris, Gallimard, 1991

On the Nature of the Psyche
in: The Basic Writings of C.G. Jung
New York: The Modern Library, 1959, 47-133

Psychological Types
Collected Writings, Vol. 6
Princeton: Princeton University Press, 1971

Psychologie und Religion
München: DTV Verlag, 2001

Psychology and Religion
in: The Basic Writings of C.G. Jung
New York: The Modern Library, 1959, 582-655

Religious and Psychological Problems of Alchemy
in: The Basic Writings of C.G. Jung
New York: The Modern Library, 1959, 537-581

Symbol und Libido
Freiburg: Walter Verlag, 1987

Synchronizität, Akausalität und Okkultismus
Frankfurt/M: DTV, 2001

The Basic Writings of C.G. Jung
New York: The Modern Library, 1959

The Development of Personality
Collected Writings, Vol. 17
Princeton: Princeton University Press, 1954

The Meaning and Significance of Dreams
Boston: Sigo Press, 1991

The Myth of the Divine Child
in: Essays on A Science of Mythology
Princeton, N.J.: Princeton University Press Bollingen
Series XXII, 1969. (With Karl Kerenyi)

Traum und Traumdeutung
München: DTV Verlag, 2001

Two Essays on Analytical Psychology
Collected Writings, Vol. 7
Princeton: Princeton University Press, 1972
First published by Routledge & Kegan Paul, Ltd., 1953

Zur Psychologie westlicher und östlicher Religion
Fünfte Auflage
Olten: Walter Verlag, 1988

K

Kahn, Charles (Ed.)
The Art and Thought of Heraclitus
Cambridge: Cambridge University Press, 2008

Kapleau, Roshi Philip
Three Pillars of Zen
Boston: Beacon Press, 1967

Karagulla, Shafica
The Chakras
Correlations between Medical Science and Clairvoyant Observation
With Dora van Gelder Kunz
Wheaton: Quest Books, 1989

Die Chakras und die feinstofflichen Körper des Menschen
Mit Dora van Gelder-Kunz
Grafing: Aquamarin Verlag, 1994

Kerner Justinus

F.A. Mesmer aus Schwaben
Frankfurt/M, 1856

Kiang, Kok Kok

The I Ching
An Illustrated Guide to the Chinese Art of Divination
Singapore: Asiapac, 1993

Kiesewetter, Carl

Franz Anton Mesmer's Leben und Lehre
Leipzig, 1893

Kingston, Karen

Creating Sacred Space With Feng Shui
New York: Broadway Books, 1997

Klimo, Jon

Channeling
Investigations on Receiving Information from Paranormal Sources
New York: North Atlantic Books, 1988

Koestler, Arthur

The Act of Creation
New York: Penguin Arkana, 1989.
Originally published in 1964

Krafft-Ebing, Richard von

Psychopathia sexualis
New York: Bell Publishing, 1965
Originally published in 1886

Krause, Donald G.

The Art of War for Executives
London: Nicholas Brealey Publishing, 1995

Krishnamurti, J.

Freedom From The Known
San Francisco: Harper & Row, 1969

The First and Last Freedom
San Francisco: Harper & Row, 1975

Education and the Significance of Life
London: Victor Gollancz, 1978

Commentaries on Living
First Series
London: Victor Gollancz, 1985

Commentaries on Living
Second Series
London: Victor Gollancz, 1986
Krishnamurti's Journal
London: Victor Gollancz, 1987

Krishnamurti's Notebook
London: Victor Gollancz, 1986

Beyond Violence
London: Victor Gollancz, 1985

Beginnings of Learning
New York: Penguin, 1986

The Penguin Krishnamurti Reader
New York: Penguin, 1987

On God
San Francisco: Harper & Row, 1992

On Fear
San Francisco: Harper & Row, 1995

The Essential Krishnamurti
San Francisco: Harper & Row, 1996

The Ending of Time
With Dr. David Bohm
San Francisco: Harper & Row, 1985

Kwok, Man-Ho

The Feng Shui Kit
London: Piatkus, 1995

L

Labate, Beatriz Caluby

Ayahuasca Religions
A Comprehensive Bibliography and Critical Essays
Santa Cruz, CA: Maps, 2009

Laing, Ronald David

Divided Self
New York: Viking Press, 1991

R.D. Laing and the Paths of Anti-Psychiatry
ed., by Z. Kotowicz
London: Routledge, 1997

The Politics of Experience
New York: Pantheon, 1983

Sagesse, déraison et folie
Paris: Seuil, 1986

Lakhovsky, Georges

La Science et le Bonheur
Longévité et Immortalité par les Vibrations
Paris: Gauthier-Villars, 1930

Le Secret de la Vie
Paris: Gauthier-Villars, 1929

Secret of Life
New York: Kessinger Publishing, 2003

L'étiologie du Cancer
Paris: Gauthier-Villars, 1929

L'Universion
Paris: Gauthier-Villars, 1927

Laszlo, Ervin

Holos. Die Welt der neuen Wissenschaften
Petersberg: Via Nova Verlag, 2002

Science and the Akashic Field
An Integral Theory of Everything
Rochester: Inner Traditions, 2004

Macroshift
Die Herausforderung
Frankfurt/M: Insel Verlag, 2003

Quantum Shift to the Global Brain
How the New Scientific Reality Can Change Us and Our World
Rochester: Inner Traditions, 2008

Science and the Reenchantment of the Cosmos
The Rise of the Integral Vision of Reality
Rochester: Inner Traditions, 2006

The Akashic Experience
Science and the Cosmic Memory Field
Rochester: Inner Traditions, 2009

The Chaos Point
The World at the Crossroads
Newburyport, MA: Hampton Roads Publishing, 2006

Leadbeater, Charles Webster

Astral Plane
Its Scenery, Inhabitants and Phenomena
Kessinger Publishing Reprint Edition, 1997

Dreams
What they Are and How they are Caused
London: Theosophical Publishing Society, 1903
Kessinger Publishing Reprint Edition, 1998

The Inner Life
Chicago: The Rajput Press, 1911
Kessinger Publishing

Leary, Timothy

Our Brain is God
Berkeley, CA: Ronin Publishing, 2001
Author Copyright 1988

Über die Kriminalisierung des Natürlichen
Löhrbach: Werner Pieper Verlag, 1990

Leboyer, Frederick

Birth Without Violence
New York, 1975

Pour une Naissance sans Violence
Paris: Seuil, 1974

Geburt ohne Gewalt
München: Kösel 1981

Cette Lumière d'où vient l'Enfant
Paris: Seuil, 1978

Inner Beauty, Inner Light
New York: Newmarket Press, 1997

Weg des Lichts
München: Kösel, 1991

Loving Hands
The Traditional Art of Baby Massage
New York: Newmarket Press, 1977

Sanfte Hände
Die Kunst der indischen Baby-Massage
München: Kösel, 1979

The Art of Breathing
New York: Newmarket Press, 1991

LeCron, Leslie M.
L'auto-hypnose
8e édition
Genève: Ariston, 1984

Leggett, Trevor P.
A First Zen Reader
Rutland: C.E. Tuttle, 1980
Originally published in 1972

Leonard, George, Murphy, Michael
The Live We Are Given
A Long Term Program for Realizing the
Potential of Body, Mind, Heart and Soul
New York: Jeremy P. Tarcher/Putnam, 1984

Liedloff, Jean
Continuum Concept
In Search of Happiness Lost
New York: Perseus Books, 1986
First published in 1977

Auf der Suche nach dem verlorenen Glück
Gegen die Zerstörung der Glücksfähigkeit in der frühen Kindheit
München: C.H. Beck Verlag, 2006

Lipton, Bruce

The Biology of Belief
Unleashing the Power of Consciousness, Matter and Miracles
Santa Rosa, CA: Mountain of Love/Elite Books, 2005

Intelligente Zellen
Wie Erfahrungen unsere Gene steuern
Burgrain: Koha Verlag, 2006

Liss, Jérôme

Débloquez vos émotions
Lausanne: Éditions Far, 1988

Long, Max *Freedom*

The Secret Science at Work
The Huna Method as a Way of Life
Marina del Rey: De Vorss Publications, 1995
Originally published in 1953

Geheimes Wissen hinter Wundern
Die Entdeckung der HUNA-Lehre
Darmstadt: Schirner Verlag, 2006

Growing Into Light
A Personal Guide to Practicing the Huna Method,
Marina del Rey: De Vorss Publications, 1955

Lowen, Alexander

Angst vor dem Leben
Über den Ursprung seelischen Leides und den Weg zu
einem reicheren Dasein
München: Goldmann Wilhelm, 1989

Bioenergetics
New York: Coward, McGoegham 1975

Bioenergetik
Therapie der Seele durch Arbeit mit dem Körper
Berlin: Rowohlt, 2008

Depression and the Body
The Biological Basis of Faith and Reality
New York: Penguin, 1992

Fear of Life
New York: Bioenergetic Press, 2003

Honoring the Body
The Autobiography of Alexander Lowen
New York: Bioenergetic Press, 2004

Joy
The Surrender to the Body and to Life
New York: Penguin, 1995

Liebe und Orgasmus
Persönlichkeitserfahrung durch sexuelle Erfüllung
München: Goldmann Wilhelm, 1993

Love and Orgasm
New York: Macmillan, 1965

Love, Sex and Your Heart
New York: Bioenergetics Press, 2004

Narcissism: Denial of the True Self
New York: Macmillan, Collier Books, 1983

Narzissmus
Die Verleugnung des wahren Selbst
München: Goldmann Wilhelm, 1992

Pleasure: A Creative Approach to Life
New York: Bioenergetics Press, 2004
First published in 1970

The Language of the Body
Physical Dynamics of Character Structure
New York: Bioenergetics Press, 2006

Lusk, Julie T. (Editor)

30 Scripts for Relaxation Imagery & Inner Healing
Whole Person Associates, 1992

Lutyens, Mary

Krishnamurti: The Years of Fulfillment
New York: Avon Books, 1983

Krishnamurti: Die Biographie
München: Aquamarin Verlag, 1997

The Life and Death of Krishnamurti
Chennai: Krishnamurti Foundation India, 1990

M

Maharshi, Ramana

The Collected Works of Ramana Maharshi
New York: Sri Ramanasramam, 2002

The Essential Teachings of Ramana Maharshi
A Visual Journey
New York: Inner Directions Publishing, 2002
by Matthew Greenblad

Sei was du bist!
München: O.W. Barth, 2001

Nan Yar? Wer bin ich?
München: Kamphausen, 2002

Maisel, Eric

Fearless Creating
A Step-By-Step Guide to Starting and Completing
Work of Art
New York: Tarcher & Putnam, 1995

Mann, Edward W.

Orgone, Reich & Eros
Wilhelm Reich's Theory of Life Energy
New York: Simon & Schuster (Touchstone), 1973

Martinson, Floyd M.

Sexual Knowledge
Values and Behavior Patterns
St. Peter: Minn.: Gustavus Adolphus College, 1966

Infant and Child Sexuality
St. Peter: Minn.: Gustavus Adolphus College, 1973

The Quality of Adolescent Experiences
St. Peter: Minn.: Gustavus Adolphus College, 1974

The Child and the Family
Calgary, Alberta: The University of Calgary, 1980

The Sex Education of Young Children
in: Lorna Brown (Ed.), *Sex Education in the Eighties*
New York, London: Plenum Press, 1981, pp. 51 ff.

The Sexual Life of Children
New York: Bergin & Garvey, 1994

Children and Sex, Part II: Childhood Sexuality
in: Bullough & Bullough, Human Sexuality (1994)
Pp. 111-116

Master Lam Kam Chuen

The Way of Energy
Mastering the Chinese Art of Internal
Strength with Chi Kung Exercise
New York: Simon & Schuster (Fireside), 1991

Master Liang, Shou-Yu & Wu, Wen-Ching

Tai Chi Chuan
24 & 48 Postures With Martial Applications
Roslindale, Mass.: YMAA Publication Center, 1996

McCarey, William A.

In Search of Healing
Whole-Body Healing Through the Mind-Body-Spirit Connection
New York: Berkley Publishing, 1996

McKenna, Terence

The Archaic Revival
San Francisco: Harper & Row, 1992

Food of The Gods
A Radical History of Plants, Drugs and Human Evolution
London: Rider, 1992

Die Speisen der Götter
Berlin: Synergia/Syntropia, 1996

The Invisible Landscape
Mind Hallucinogens and the I Ching
New York: HarperCollins, 1993
(With Dennis McKenna)

True Hallucinations
Being the Account of the Author's Extraordinary
Adventures in the Devil's Paradise
New York: Fine Communications, 1998

McNiff, Shaun

Art as Medicine
Boston: Shambhala, 1992

Art as Therapy
Creating a Therapy of the Imagination
Boston/London: Shambhala, 1992

Trust the Process
An Artist's Guide to Letting Go
New York: Shambhala Publications, 1998

McTaggart, Lynne

The Field
The Quest for the Secret Force of the Universe
New York: Harper & Collins, 2002

Mead, Margaret

Sex and Temperament in Three Primitive Societies
New York, 1935

Meadows, Donella H.

Thinking in Systems
A Primer
White River, VT: Chelsea Green Publishing, 2008

Mehta, Rohit

J. Krishnamurti and the Nameless Experience
A Comprehensive Discussion of J. Krishnamurti's Approach to Life
Delhi: Motilal Banarsidass Publishers, 2002

Méric, de, Philippe

Le Yoga sans postures
Paris: Livre de Poche, 1967

Merleau-Ponty, Maurice

Phenomenology of Perception
London: Routledge, 1995
Originally published 1945

Phénoménologie de la perception
Paris: Gallimard, 1945

Metzner, Ralph (Ed.)

Ayahuasca, Human Consciousness and the Spirits of Nature
ed. by Ralph Metzner, Ph.D
New York: Thunder's Mouth Press, 1999

The Psychedelic Experience
A Manual Based on the Tibetan Book of the Dead
With Timothy Leary and Richard Alpert
New York: Citadel, 1995

Miller, Alice

Four Your Own Good
Hidden Cruelty in Child-Rearing and the Roots of Violence
New York: Farrar, Straus & Giroux, 1983

Am Anfang war Erziehung
München: Suhrkamp Verlag, 2008
Erstmals publiziert im Jahre 1986

Pictures of a Childhood
New York: Farrar, Straus & Giroux, 1986

The Drama of the Gifted Child
In Search for the True Self
translated by Ruth Ward
New York: Basic Books, 1996

Das Drama des Begabten Kindes
Und die Suche nach dem wahren Selbst
München: Suhrkamp Verlag, 1983

Der gemiedene Schlüssel
München: Suhrkamp, 2007

Das verbannte Wissen
Frankfurt/M: Suhrkamp, 1988

Thou Shalt Not Be Aware
Society's Betrayal of the Child
New York: Noonday, 1998

Du Sollst Nicht Merken
Variationen über das Paradies-Thema
Neuauflage
München: Suhrkamp, 2005

The Political Consequences of Child Abuse
in: The Journal of Psychohistory 26, 2 (Fall 1998)

Moll, Albert

The Sexual Life of the Child
New York: Macmillan, 1912
First published in German as
Das Sexualleben des Kindes, 1909

Monroe, Robert

Ultimate Journey
New York: Broadway Books, 1994

Montagu, Ashley

Touching
The Human Significance of the Skin
New York: Harper & Row, 1978

Körperkontakt
8. Auflage
Stuttgart: Klett/Cotta, 1995

Montessori, Maria

The Absorbent Mind
Reprint Edition
New York: Buccaneer Books, 1995
First published in 1973

Das Kreative Kind
Der absorbierende Geist
Freiburg: Herder, 2007

Moody, Raymond

The Light Beyond
New York: Mass Market Paperback (Bantam), 1989

Moore, Thomas

Care of the Soul
A Guide for Cultivating Depth and Sacredness in Everyday Life
New York: Harper & Collins, 1994

Die Seele Lieben
Tiefe und Spiritualität im täglichen Leben
München: Droemer Knaur, 1995

Murphy, Joseph

The Power of Your Subconscious Mind
West Nyack, N.Y.: Parker, 1981, N.Y.: Bantam, 1982
Originally published in 1962

Die Macht Ihres Unterbewusstseins
München: Hugendubel, 2000

La puissance de votre subconscient
Genève: Ramón Keller, 1967

The Miracle of Mind Dynamics
New York: Prentice Hall, 1964

Miracle Power for Infinite Riches
West Nyack, N.Y.: Parker, 1972

The Amazing Laws of Cosmic Mind Power
West Nyack, N.Y.: Parker, 1973

Secrets of the I Ching
West Nyack, N.Y.: Parker, 1970

Think Yourself Rich
Use the Power of Your Subconscious Mind to Find True Wealth
Revised by Ian D. McMahan, Ph.D.
Paramus, NJ: Reward Books, 2001

Wahrheiten die ihr Leben verändern
Dr. Joseph Murphys Vermächtnis
München: Hugendubel, 1996

Murphy, Michael

The Future of the Body
Explorations into the Further Evolution of Human Nature
New York: Jeremy P. Tarcher/Putnam, 1992

Der Quanten-Mensch
München: Ludwig Verlag, 1996

Myers, Tony Pearce

The Soul of Creativity
Insights into the Creative Process
Novato, CA: New World Library, 1999

Myss, Caroline

The Creation of Health
The Emotional, Psychological, and Spiritual Responses that Promote
Health and Healing
New York: Three Rivers Press, 1998

N

Naparstek, Belleruth

Your Sixth Sense
Unlocking the Power of Your Intuition
London: HarperCollins, 1998

Staying Well With Guided Imagery
New York: Warner Books, 1995

Narby, Jeremy

The Cosmic Serpent
DNA and the Origins of Knowledge
New York: J. P. Tarcher, 1999

Die Kosmische Schlange
Auf den Pfaden der Schamanen zu den Ursprüngen modernen Wissens
Stuttgart: Klett-Cotta, 2007

Nau, Erika

Self-Awareness Through Huna
Virginia Beach: Donning, 1981

Selbstbewusst durch Huna
Die magische Weisheit Hawaiis
2. Auflage
Basel: Sphinx Verlag, 1989

Neumann, Erich

The Great Mother
Princeton: Princeton University Press, 1955
(Bollingen Series)

Die Grosse Mutter
Die weiblichen Gestaltungen des Unterbewussten
Düsseldorf: Patmos Verlag, 2003

Newton, Michael

Life Between Lives
Hypnotherapy for Spiritual Regression
Woodbury, Minn.: Llewellyn Publications, 2006

Ni, Hua-Ching

I Ching
The Book of Changes and the Unchanging Truth
2nd edition
Santa Barbara: Seven Star Communications, 1999

Esoteric Tao The Ching
The Shrine of the Eternal Breath of Tao
Santa Monica: College of Tao and Traditional
Chinese Healing, 1992

The Complete Works of Lao Tzu
Tao The Ching & Hua Hu Ching
Translation and Elucidation by Hua-Ching Ni
Santa Monica: Seven Star Communications, 1995

Nichols, Sallie

Jung and Tarot: An Archetypal Journey
New York: Red Wheel/Weiser, 1986

Die Psychologie des Tarot
Interlaken: Ansata Verlag, 1996

O

Odent, Michel

Birth Reborn
What Childbirth Should Be
London: Souvenir Press, 1994

The Scientification of Love
London: Free Association Books, 1999

Die Wurzeln der Liebe
Wie unsere wichtigsten Emotionen entstehen
Olten: Walter Verlag, 2001

Primal Health
Understanding the Critical Period Between Conception
and the First Birthday
London: Clairview Books, 2002
First Published in 1986 with Century Hutchinson in London

La Santé Primale
Paris: Payot, 1986

Die sanfte Geburt
Die Leboyer-Methode in der Praxis
Bergisch-Gladbach: Lübbe Verlag, 2001

The Functions of the Orgasms
The Highway to Transcendence
London: Pinter & Martin, 2009

Ong, Hean-Tatt

Amazing Scientific Basis of Feng-Shui
Kuala Lumpur: Eastern Dragon Press, 1997

Ostrander, Sheila & Schroeder, Lynn

Superlearning 2000
New York: Delacorte Press, 1994

Superlearning
Die revolutionäre Lernmethode
München: Scherz Verlag, 1979

Supermemory
New York: Carroll & Graf, 1991

SuperMemory
Der Weg zum optimalen Gedächtnis
München: Goldmann, 1996

Ouspensky, Pyotr Demianovich

In Search of the Miraculous
New York: Mariner Books, 2001
First published in 1949

P

Pearce Myers, Tony (Editor)

The Soul of Creativity
Insights into the Creative Process
Novato: New World Library, 1999

Pert, Candace B.

Molecules of Emotion
The Science Behind Mind-Body Medicine
New York: Scribner, 2003

Petrash, Jack

Understanding Waldorf Education
Teaching from the Inside Out
London: Floris Books, 2003

Ponder, Catherine

The Healing Secrets of the Ages
Marine del Rey: DeVorss, 1985

Porteous, Hedy S.

Sex and Identity
Your Child's Sexuality
Indianapolis: Bobbs-Merrill, 1972

R

Radin, Dean

The Conscious Universe
The Scientific Truth of Psychic Phenomena
San Francisco: Harper & Row, 1997

Entangled Minds
Extrasensory Experiences in a Quantum Reality
New York: Paraview Pocket Books, 2006

Raknes, Ola

Wilhelm Reich and Orgonomy
Oslo: Universitetsforlaget, 1970

Wilhelm Reich und die Orgonomie
Eine Einführung in die Wissenschaft von der Lebensenergie
Frankfurt/M: Nexus, 1983

Randall, Neville

Life After Death
London: Robert Hale, 1999

Rank, Otto

Art and Artist
With Charles Francis Atkinson and Anaïs Nin
New York: W.W. Norton, 1989
Originally published in 1932

The Significance of Psychoanalysis for the Mental Sciences
New York: BiblioBazaar, 2009
First published in 1913

Rausky, Franklin

Mesmer ou la révolution thérapeutique
Paris, 1977

Redfield, James

The Tenth Insight
Holding the Vision
New York: Warner Books, 1996

The Celestine Prophecy
New York: Warner Books, 1995

Die Vision von Celestine
Berlin: Ullstein, 2004

Reich, Wilhelm

A Review of the Theories, dating from The 17th Century,
on the Origin of Organic Life
by Arthur Hahn, Literature Assistant at the Institut für
Sexualökonomische Lebensforschung, Biologisches Laboratorium,
Oslo, 1938
©1979 Mary Boyd Higgins as Director of the Wilhelm Reich Infant Trust
XEROX Copy from the Wilhelm Reich Museum

Children of the Future
On the Prevention of Sexual Pathology
New York: Farrar, Straus & Giroux, 1984
First published in 1950

CORE (Cosmic Orgone Engineering)
Part I, Space Ships, DOR and DROUGHT
©1984, Orgone Institute Press
XEROX Copy from the Wilhelm Reich Museum

Der Einbruch der sexuellen Zwangsmoral
Frankfurt/M: Fischer, 1981

Die Entdeckung des Orgons II
Der Krebs
Frankfurt/M: Fischer, 1981
Köln: Kiepenheuer & Witsch, 1984

Die Funktion des Orgasmus

Sexualökonomische Grundprobleme der biologischen Energie
Köln: Kiepenheuer & Witsch, 1987

Die Massenpsychologie des Faschismus
Frankfurt/M: Fischer, 1974

Die sexuelle Revolution
Frankfurt/M: Fischer, 1966

Early Writings 1
New York: Farrar, Straus & Giroux, 1975

Ether, God & Devil & Cosmic Superimposition
New York: Farrar, Straus & Giroux, 1972
Originally published in 1949

Frühe Schriften 1
Aus den Jahren 1920-1925
Frankfurt/M: Fischer, 1983

Frühe Schriften 2
Genitalität in der Theorie und Therapie der Neurose
Frankfurt/M: Fischer, 1985

Genitality in the Theory and Therapy of Neurosis
©1980 by Mary Boyd Higgins as Director of the Wilhelm Reich
Infant Trust

Leidenschaften der Jugend
Köln: Kiepenheuer & Witsch, 1984

L'irruption de la morale sexuelle
Paris: Payot, 1972

Menschen im Staat
Frankfurt/M: Nexus, 1982

People in Trouble
©1974 by Mary Boyd Higgins as Director of the Wilhelm Reich
Infant Trust

Record of a Friendship
The Correspondence of Wilhelm Reich and A. S. Neill
New York, Farrar, Straus & Giroux, 1981

Selected Writings
An Introduction to Orgonomy
New York: Farrar, Straus & Giroux, 1973

The Bioelectrical Investigation of Sexuality and Anxiety
New York: Farrar, Straus & Giroux, 1983
Originally published in 1935

The Bion Experiments
reprinted in *Selected Writings*
New York: Farrar, Straus & Giroux, 1973

The Cancer Biopathy (The Orgone, Vol. 2)
New York: Farrar, Straus & Giroux, 1973

The Function of the Orgasm (The Orgone, Vol. 1)
Orgone Institute Press, New York, 1942

The Invasion of Compulsory Sex Morality
New York: Farrar, Straus & Giroux, 1971
Originally published in 1932

The Leukemia Problem: Approach
©1951, Orgone Institute Press
Copyright Renewed 1979
XEROX Copy from the Wilhelm Reich Museum

The Mass Psychology of Fascism
New York: Farrar, Straus & Giroux, 1970
Originally published in 1933

The Orgone Energy Accumulator
Its Scientific and Medical Use
©1951, 1979, Orgone Institute Press
XEROX Copy from the Wilhelm Reich Museum

The Schizophrenic Split
©1945, 1949, 1972 by Mary Boyd Higgins as Director of the
Wilhelm Reich Infant Trust
XEROX Copy from the Wilhelm Reich Museum

The Sexual Revolution
©1945, 1962 by Mary Boyd Higgins as Director of the
Wilhelm Reich Infant Trust

Zeugnisse einer Freundschaft
Der Briefwechsel zwischen Wilhelm Reich und A.S.
Neill (1936-1957)
Köln: Kiepenheuer & Witsch, 1986

Reid, Daniel P.

The Tao of Health, Sex & Longevity
A Modern Practical Guide to the Ancient Way
New York: Simon & Schuster, 1989

Guarding the Three Treasures
The Chinese Way of Health
New York: Simon & Schuster, 1993

Reps, Paul

Zen Flesh, Zen Bones
Rutland: Tuttle Publishing, 1989

Riso, Don Richard & Hudson, Russ

The Wisdom of the Enneagram
The Complete Guide to Psychological and Spiritual Growth
For The Nine Personality Types
New York: Bantam Books, 1999

Robbins, Anthony

Awaken The Giant Within
New York: Simon & Schuster, 1991

Unlimited Power
The New Science of Personal Achievement
New York: Free Press, 1997

Roberts, Jane

The Nature of Personal Reality
New York: Amber-Allen Publishing, 1994
First published in 1974

Die Natur der Persönlichen Realität
Ein neues Bewusstsein als Quelle der Kreativität
München: Kailash Verlag, 2007

The Nature of the Psyche
Its Human Expression
New York, Amber-Allen Publishing, 1996
First published in 1979

Die Natur der Psyche
Ihr menschlicher Ausdruck in Kreativität, Liebe, Sexualität
Genf: Ariston Verlag, 1985

Die Natur der Psyche
Ihr menschlicher Ausdruck in Kreativität, Liebe, Sexualität
München: Kailash Verlag, 2008

Roman, Sanaya

Opening to Channel
How To Connect With Your Guide
New York: H.J. Kramer, 1987

Zum Höheren Selbst Erwachen
Das Herz dem Bewusstsein des Lichts öffnen
Genf: Ansata Verlag, 2003

Rosen, Sydney (Ed.)

My Voice Will Go With You
The Teaching Tales of Milton H. Erickson
New York: Norton & Co., 1991

Rudhyar, Dane

Astrology of Personality
A Reformulation of Astrological Concepts and Ideals in
Terms of Contemporary Psychology and Philosophy
New York: Aurora Press, 1990

An Astrological Triptych
Gifts of the Spirit, The Way Through, and The Illumined Road
New York: Aurora Press, 1991

Astrological Mandala
New York: Vintage Books, 1994

L'astrologie de la transformation
Paris: Rocher, 1984

Ruiz, Don Miguel

The Four Agreements
A Practical Guide to Personal Freedom
San Rafael, CA: Amber Allen Publishing, 1997

The Mastery of Love
A Practical Guide to the Art of Relationship
San Rafael, CA: Amber Allen Publishing, 1999

The Voice of Knowledge
A Practical Guide to Inner Peace
With Janet Mills
San Rafael, CA: Amber Allen Publishing, 2004

Ruperti, Alexander

Cycles of Becoming
The Planetary Pattern of Growth
New York: CRCS Publications, 1978

La roue de l'expérience individuelle
Paris: Librairie de Médicis, 1991

S

SantoPietro, Nancy

Feng Shui, Harmony by Design
How to Create a Beautiful and Harmonious Home,
New York: Putnam-Berkeley, 1996

Satinover, Jeffrey

The Quantum Brain
New York: Wiley & Sons, 2001

Schultes, Richard Evans, et al.

Plants of the Gods
Their Sacred, Healing, and Hallucinogenic Powers
New York: Healing Arts Press
2nd edition, 2002

Die Pflanzen der Götter
Die magischen Kräfte der Rausch- und Giftgewächse
München: AT Verlag, 1998

Schwartz, Andrew E.

Guided Imagery for Groups
Fifty Visualizations That Promote Relaxation, Problem-Solving,
Creativity, and Well-Being
Whole Person Associates, 1995

Senf, Bernd

Die Wiederentdeckung des Lebendigen
Aachen: Omega, 2003
Erstmals veröffentlicht 1996 mit Zweitausendeins Verlag in Frankfurt/M

Nach Reich: Neue Forschungen zur Orgonenergie
Sexualökonomie / Die Entdeckung der Orgonenergie
Herausgegeben zusammen mit Professor James DeMeo
Frankfurt/M: Zweitausendeins Verlag, 1997

Sheldrake, Rupert

A New Science of Life
The Hypothesis of Morphic Resonance
Rochester: Park Street Press, 1995

Das Schöpferische Universum
Die Theorie des morphogenetischen Feldes
Neue und erweiterte Auflage
Berlin: Ullstein, 2009

Sher, Barbara & Gottlieb, Annie

Wishcraft
How to Get What You Really Want
2nd edition
New York: Ballantine Books, 2003

Shone, Ronald

Creative Visualization
Using Imagery and Imagination for Self-Transformation
New York: Destiny Books, 1998

Simonton, O. Carl et al.

Getting Well Again
Los Angeles: Tarcher, 1978

Singer, June

Androgyny
New York: Doubleday Dell, 1976

Smith, C. Michael

Jung and Shamanism in Dialogue
London: Trafford Publishing, 2007

Spiller, Jan

Astrology for the Soul
New York: Bantam, 1997

Spock, Benjamin

Dr. Spock's Baby and Child Care
8th Edition
New York: Pocket Books, 2004

Säuglings- und Kinderpflege
Berlin: Ullstein, 1986

Spretnak, Charlene

Green Politics
Rochester, VT: Inner Traditions, 1986

Stein, Robert M.

Redeeming the Inner Child in Marriage and Therapy
in: Reclaiming the Inner Child
ed. by Jeremiah Abrams
New York: Tarcher/Putnam, 1990, 261 ff.

Steiner, Rudolf

Theosophy
An Introduction to the Spiritual Processes in Human Life
and in the Cosmos
New York: Anthroposophic Press, 1994

Die Erziehung des Kindes
Dornach: Rudolf Steiner Verlag, 2003
First published in 1907

Stiene, Bronwen & Frans

The Reiki Sourcebook
New York: O Books, 2003

The Japanese Art of Reiki
A Practical Guide to Self-Healing
New York: O Books, 2005

Stone, Hal & Stone, Sidra

Embracing Our Selves
The Voice Dialogue Manual
San Rafael, CA: New World Library, 1989

Du bist viele
Das 100fache Selbst und seine Entdeckung durch
die Voice-Dialogue Methode
München: Heyne Verlag, 1994

Strassman, Rick

DMT: The Spirit Molecule
A doctor's revolutionary research into the biology of near-death
and mystical experiences
Rochester: Park Street Press, 2001

Sun Tzu (Sun Tsu)

The Art of War
Special Edition
New York: El Paso Norte Press, 2007

Die Kunst des Krieges
Hamburg: Nikol Verlag, 2008

Szasz, Thomas

The Myth of Mental Illness
New York: Harper & Row, 1984

T

Talbot, Michael

The Holographic Universe
New York: HarperCollins, 1992

Das holographische Universum
Die Welt in neuer Dimension
München: Droemer Knaur, 1994

Tansley, David V.

Chakras, Rays and Radionics
London: Daniel Company Ltd., 1984

Targ, Russell & Katra, Jane

Miracles of Mind
Exploring Nonlocal Consciousness and Spiritual Healing
Novato, CA: New World Library, 1999

Tarnas, Richard

Cosmos and Psyche
Intimations of a New World View
New York: Plume, 2007

The Passion of the Western Mind
Understanding the Ideas that have Shaped Our World View
New York: Ballantine Books, 1993

Tart, Charles T.

Altered States of Consciousness
A Book of Readings
Hoboken, N.J.: Wiley & Sons, 1969

Tatar, Maria M.

Spellbound: Studies on Mesmerism and Literature
Princeton, N.Y., 1978

Tchouang-tseu

Oeuvre complète
Paris: Gallimard/Unesco, 1969

Tiller, William A.

Conscious Acts of Creation
The Emergence of a New Physics
Associated Producers, 2004 (DVD)

Psychoenergetic Science
New York: Pavior, 2007

Conscious Acts of Creation
New York: Pavior, 2001

Tischner, Rudolf

F.A. Mesmer
München, 1928

Todaro-Franceschi, Vidette

The Enigma of Energy
Where Science and Religion Converge
New York: Crossroad Publishing, 1991

Tolle, Eckhart

The Power of Now
A Guide to Spiritual Enlightenment
Novato, CA: New World Library, 2004

Jetzt! Die Kraft der Gegenwart
Ein Leitfaden zum spirituellen Erwachen
Bielefeld: Kamphausen Verlag, 2000

A New Earth
Awakening to Your Life's Purpose
New York: Michael Joseph (Penguin), 2005

Eine neue Erde
Bewusstseinssprung anstelle von Selbstzerstörung
München: Goldmann, 2005

Too, Lillian

Feng Shui
Kuala Lumpur: Konsep Books, 1994

V

Villoldo, Alberto

Healing States
A Journey Into the World of Spiritual Healing and Shamanism
With Stanley Krippner
New York: Simon & Schuster (Fireside), 1987

Dance of the Four Winds
Secrets of the Inca Medicine Wheel
With Eric Jendresen
Rochester: Destiny Books, 1995

Die Macht der vier Winde
Eine Reise ins Reich der Schamanen
München: Goldmann, 2009

Shaman, Healer, Sage
How to Heal Yourself and Others with the Energy Medicine
of the Americas
New York: Harmony, 2000

Hüter des alten Wissens
Schamanisches Heilen im Medizinrad
Darmstadt: Schirner Verlag, 2007

Healing the Luminous Body
The Way of the Shaman with Dr. Alberto Villoldo
DVD, Sacred Mysteries Productions, 2004

Mending The Past And Healing The Future with Soul Retrieval
New York: Hay House, 2005

Seelenrückholung: die Vergangenheit schamanistisch erkunden
Die Zukunft heilen
München, Goldmann, 2006

W

Watts, Alan W.

The Way of Zen
New York: Vintage Books, 1999

This Is It
And Other Essays on Zen and Spiritual Experience
New York: Vintage, 1973

Wee Chow Hou

The 36 Strategies of the Chinese
Adapting Ancient Chinese Wisdom to the Business World
New York: Addison-Wesley, 2007

Whitfield, Charles L.

Healing the Child Within
Deerfield Beach, Fl: Health Communications, 1987

Wilber, Ken

Sex, Ecology, Spirituality
The Spirit of Evolution
Boston: Shambhala, 2000

Quantum Questions
Mystical Writings of The World's Greatest Physicists
Boston: Shambhala, 2001

Wilhelm, Helmut

The Wilhelm Lectures on the Book of Changes
Princeton: Princeton University Press, 1995

Wilhelm, Richard

The I Ching or Book of Changes
With C. Baynes
3rd Edition, Bollingen Series XIX
Princeton, NJ: Princeton University Press, 1967

Williams, Strephon Kaplan

Dreams and Spiritual Growth
With Patricia H. Berne and Louis M. Savary
New York: Paulist Press, 1984

Durch Traumarbeit zum eigenen Selbst
Die Jung-Senoi Methode
Interlaken: Ansata Verlag, 1987

Dream Cards
Understand Your Dreams and Enrich Your Life
New York: Simon & Schuster (Fireside), 1991

Wing, R. L.

The I Ching Workbook
Garden City, N.Y.: Doubleday, 1984

Das Arbeitsbuch zum I Ching
Mit Chinesischen Orakel Münzen
München: Goldmann, 2004

Het I Tjing Werkboek
Baarn: Bigot & Van Rossum, 1986

Woerly, Franz

Esprit Guide
Entretiens avec Karlfried Dürckheim
Paris: Albin Michel, 1985

Wolf, Fred Alan

Taking the Quantum Leap
The New Physics for Nonscientists
New York: Harper & Row, 1989

Der Quantensprung ist keine Hexerei
Frankfurt/M: Fischer Verlag, 1990

Parallel Universes
New York: Simon & Schuster, 1990

The Dreaming Universe
A Mind-Expanding Journey into the Realm Where
Psyche and Physics Meet
New York: Touchstone, 1995

The Eagle's Quest
A Physicist Finds the Scientific Truth At the Heart of the
Shamanic World
New York: Touchstone, 1997

Die Physik der Träume
Frankfurt/M: DTV Verlag, 1997

Mind into Matter
A New Alchemy of Science and Spirit
New York: Moment Point Press, 2000

Y

Yang, Jwing-Ming

Qigong, The Secret of Youth
Da Mo's Muscle/Tendon Changing and Marrow/Brain Washing Classics
Boston, Mass.: YMAA Publication Center, 2000

The Root of Chinese Qigong
Secrets for Health, Longevity, & Enlightenment
Roslindale, MA: YMAA Publication Center, 1997

Yates, Alayne

Sex Without Shame
Encouraging the Child's Healthy Sexual Development
New York, 1978
Republished Internet Edition

Ywahoo, Dhyani

Voices of Our Ancestors
Cherokee Teachings from the Wisdom Fire
New York: Shambhala, 1987

Am Feuer der Weisheit
Lehren der Cherokee Indianer
Zürich: Theseus Verlag, 1988

Z

Znamenski, Andrei A.

Shamanism
Critical Concepts in Sociology
New York: Routledge, 2004

Zinker, Joseph

Se créer par la Gestalt
Montréal: Les Éditions de l'Homme, 1981

Zukav, Gary

The Dancing Wu Li Masters
An Overview of the New Physics
New York: HarperOne, 2001

Die tanzenden Wu Li Meister
Der östliche Pfad zum Verständnis der modernen Physik
Vom Quantensprung zum schwarzen Loch
Berlin: Rowohlt, 2000

Zweig, Stefan

Die Heilung durch den Geist
Mesmer, Mary Baker-Eddy, Freud
Frankfurt/M: Fischer Verlag, 1982
Originally published in 1931

FROM THE SAME AUTHOR

A Bibliography

You can search publications from here:
http://ipublica.com/books/

For audio books and music, you can start here:
http://ipublica.com/audio/

All paperbacks, audio downloads, audio book compact discs, music downloads and music compact discs, as well as Kindle books, are referenced on the site, ipublica.com.

For free podcasts search iTunes under my author name.

For quoting my publications, please use the following form:
Pierre F. Walter, [Title]: [Subtitle], Newark: Sirius-C Media Galaxy LLC, 2011

Web Presence

Pierre F. Walter on the Web

Sites

http://authoryourlife.com

http://ipublica.com

http://ipublica.net

http://ipublica.org

http://ipublica.tv

Video Channels

http://youtube.com/user/ipublica

http://youtube.com/user/authoryourlife

http://vimeo.com/pierrefwalter/channels

http://ipublica.blip.tv/

http://authoryourlife.blip.tv/

http://emosexuality.blip.tv/

http://pierrefwalter.blip.tv/